101 DESCRIPTIVE WORDS

FOR FOOD EXPLORERS

A Visual Guide for
Adventures in Food

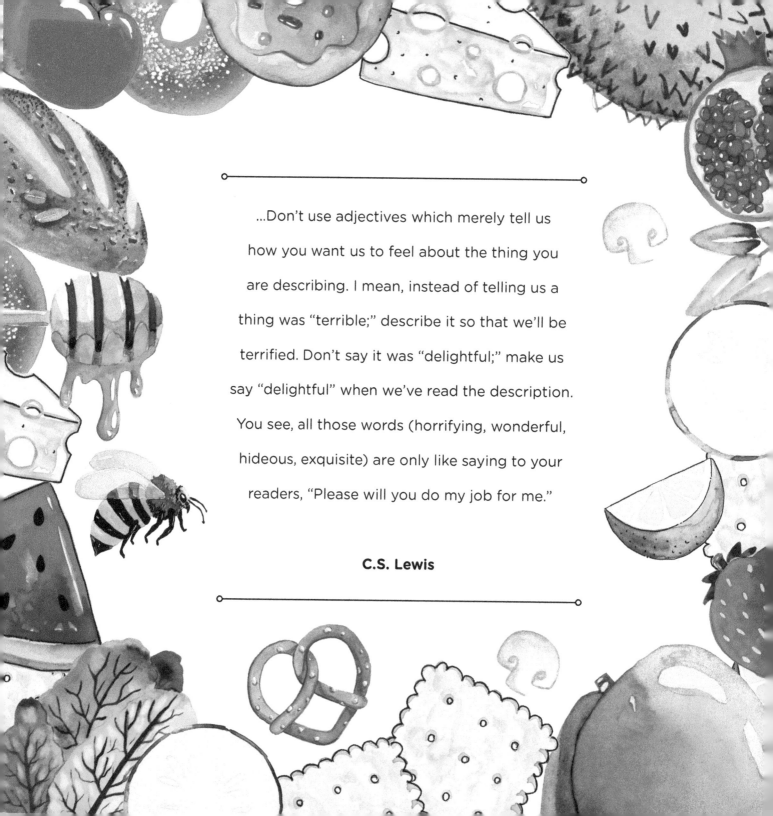

...Don't use adjectives which merely tell us how you want us to feel about the thing you are describing. I mean, instead of telling us a thing was "terrible;" describe it so that we'll be terrified. Don't say it was "delightful;" make us say "delightful" when we've read the description. You see, all those words (horrifying, wonderful, hideous, exquisite) are only like saying to your readers, "Please will you do my job for me."

C.S. Lewis

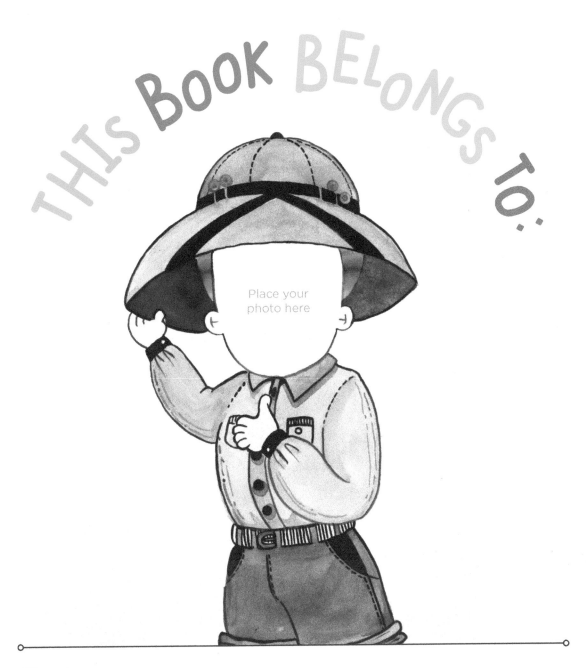

THIS BOOK BELONGS TO:

Place your
photo here

FOOD EXPLORER:

Write your name above

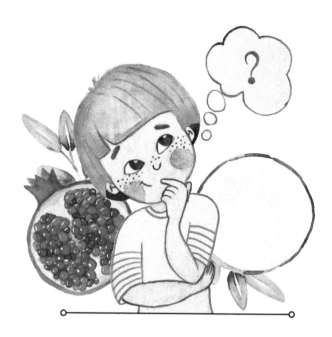

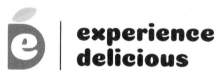

experience delicious

Experience Delicious LLC

Copyright 2020 Experience Delicious, LLC.
ISBN: 978-1-947001-26-8
www.experiencedeliciousnow.com

WELCOME!
FOOD EXPLORER

How would you tell someone about your favorite toy or stuffed animal if they have never seen it or played with it before? Would you tell them the color, size, or shape? Would you compare it to another toy they may have seen?

All the words we use to describe something are called adjectives or descriptive words. Descriptive words help us better explain what we are trying to communicate.

Learning descriptive words is important when exploring foods because it helps us understand what we like and dislike about them. Sometimes we learn about new flavors, textures, or even different ways to prepare foods. Descriptive words help us better share our food preferences, or what we like about certain foods, so we can continue to be adventurous and try new things.

Let this book help guide your taste buds as you increase your vocabulary and expand your favorite food list.

Now put your Food Explorer hat on and let's search for delicious!

TABLE OF CONTENTS

MY FIVE SENSES

We can explore anything using our five senses. Exploring food with our five senses is fun and can help us discover and connect with what we eat. Our five senses send information to our brain about the look, feel, smell, sound, and taste of a food. Learning and using descriptive words is a tool that helps us understand qualities about foods and explain what we like or dislike about them.

sEE

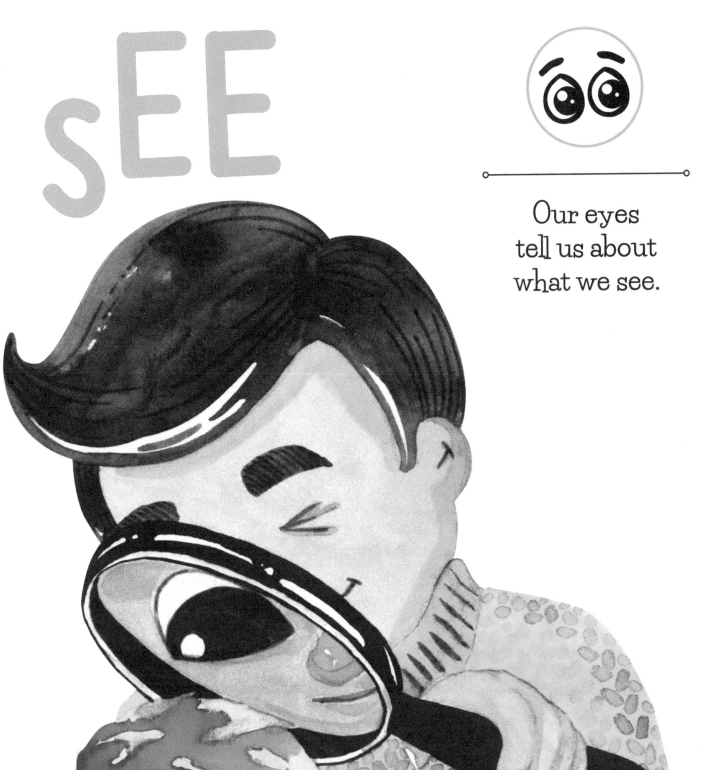

Our eyes
tell us about
what we see.

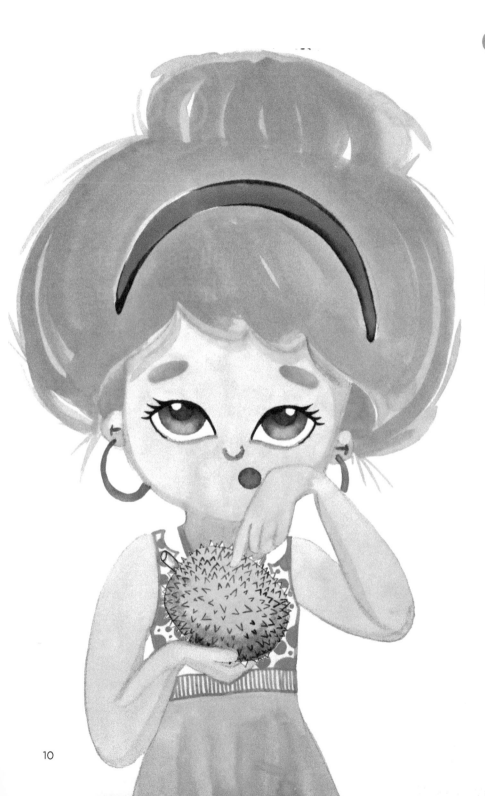

TOUCH

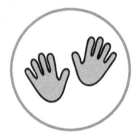

Our hands and
mouth tell us about
the textures
we feel.

SMELL

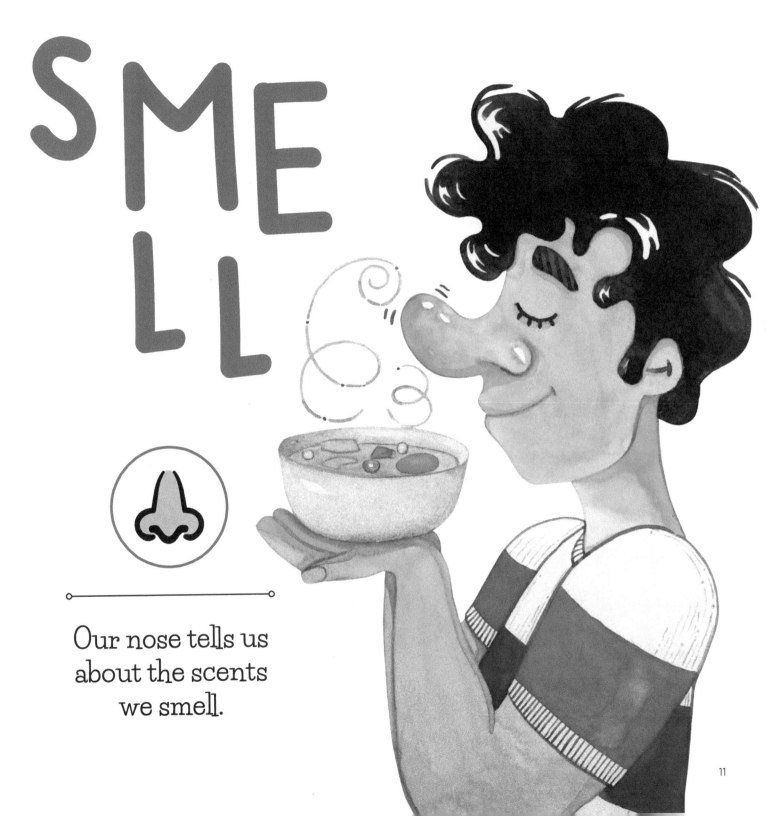

Our nose tells us about the scents we smell.

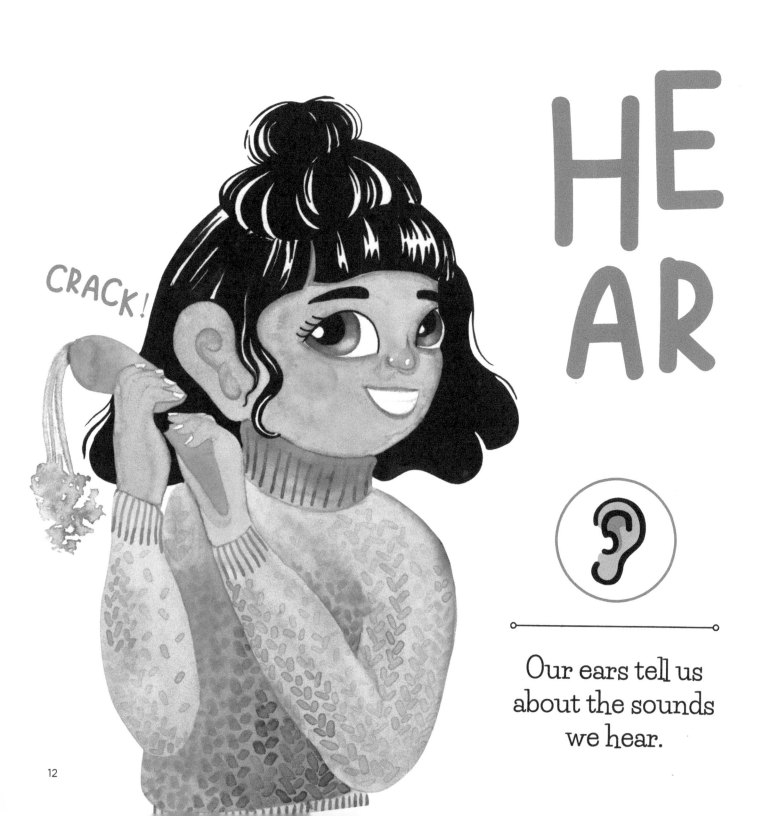

CRACK!

HE
AR

Our ears tell us
about the sounds
we hear.

12

TASTE

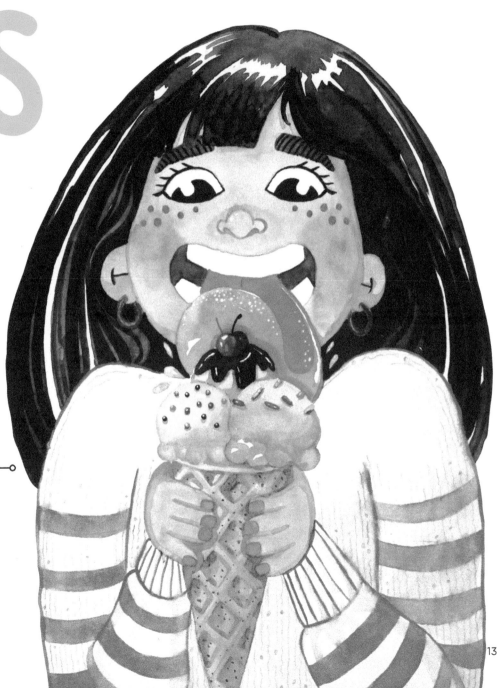

Our tongue
tells us about
the flavors
we taste.

ACIDIC

bitter, sharp, sour

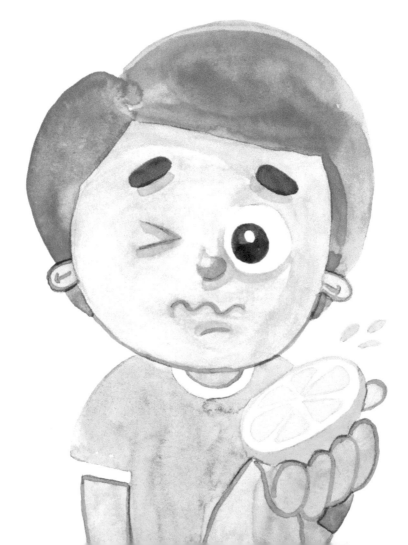

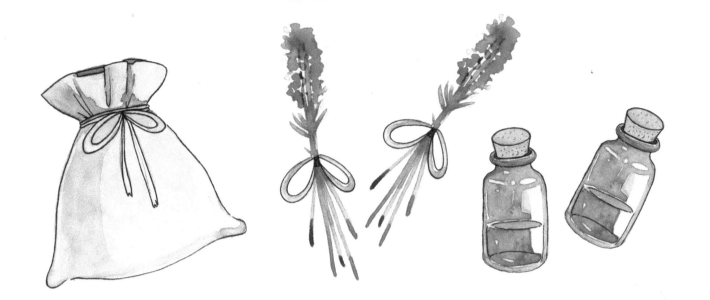

AROMATIC

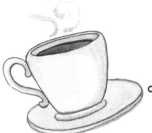

good scent, smell, odor

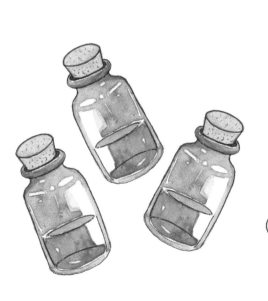

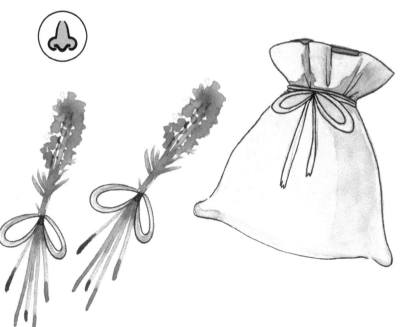

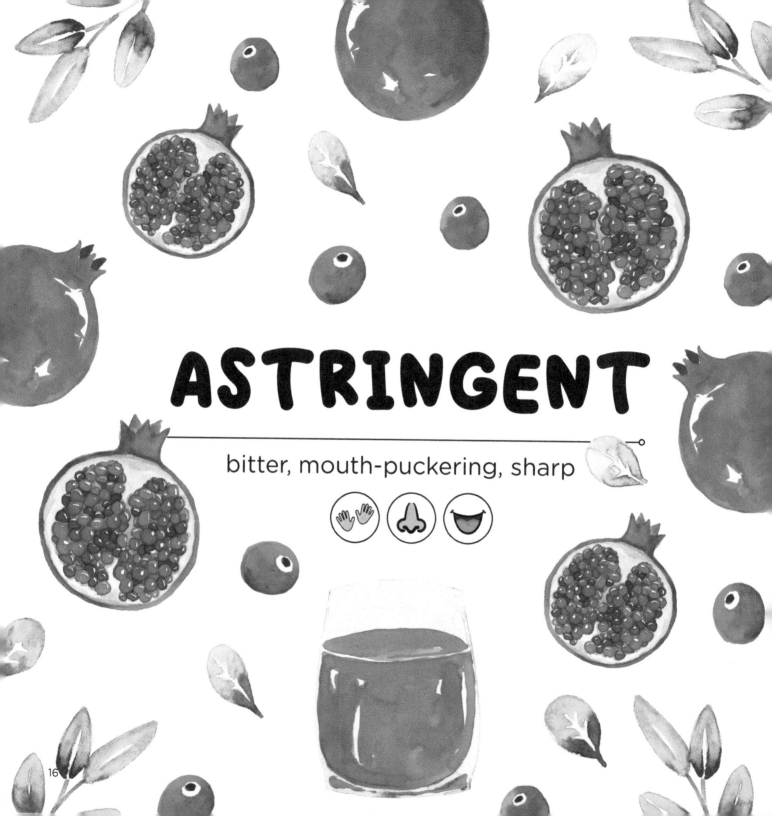

ASTRINGENT

bitter, mouth-puckering, sharp

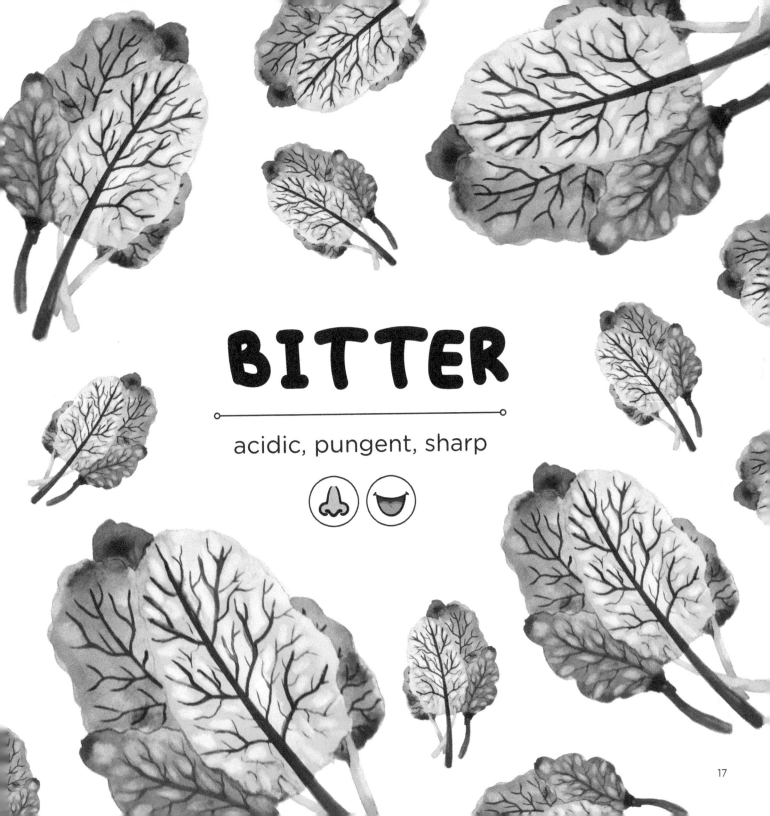

BITTER

acidic, pungent, sharp

BLAND

flavorless, mild, tasteless

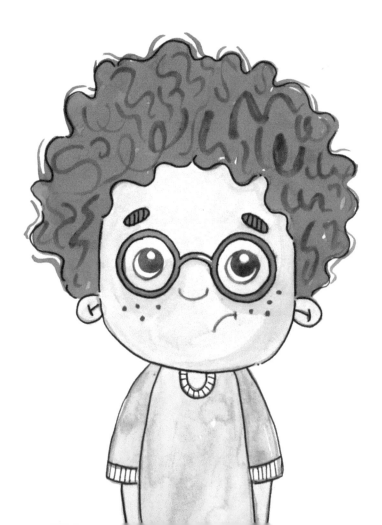

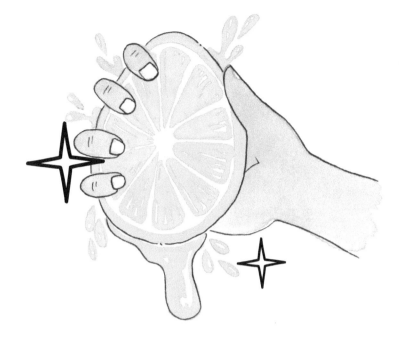

BRIGHT

acidic, fresh, sharp,
strong color, full of light

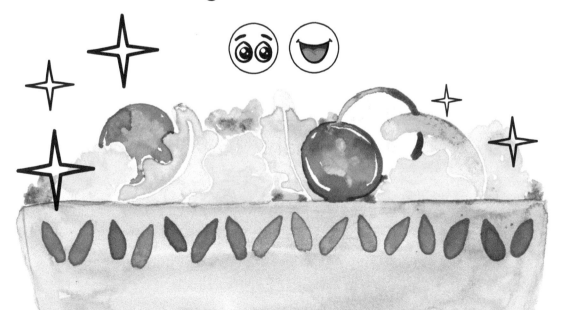

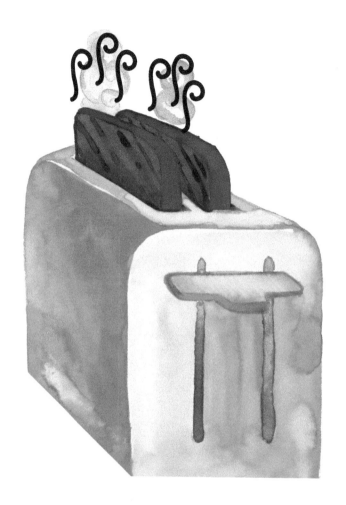

BURNT

charred, crunchy, overcooked

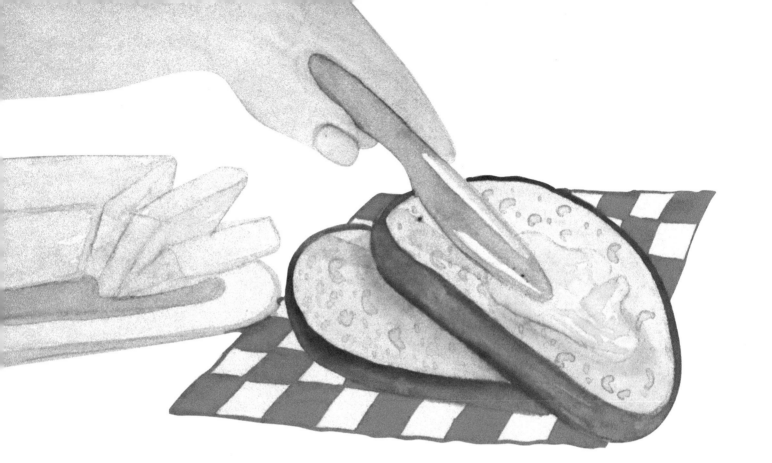

BUTTERY

creamy, rich, smooth,
looks, feels, smells, or tastes
similar to butter

CHEWY

leathery, rubbery, tough

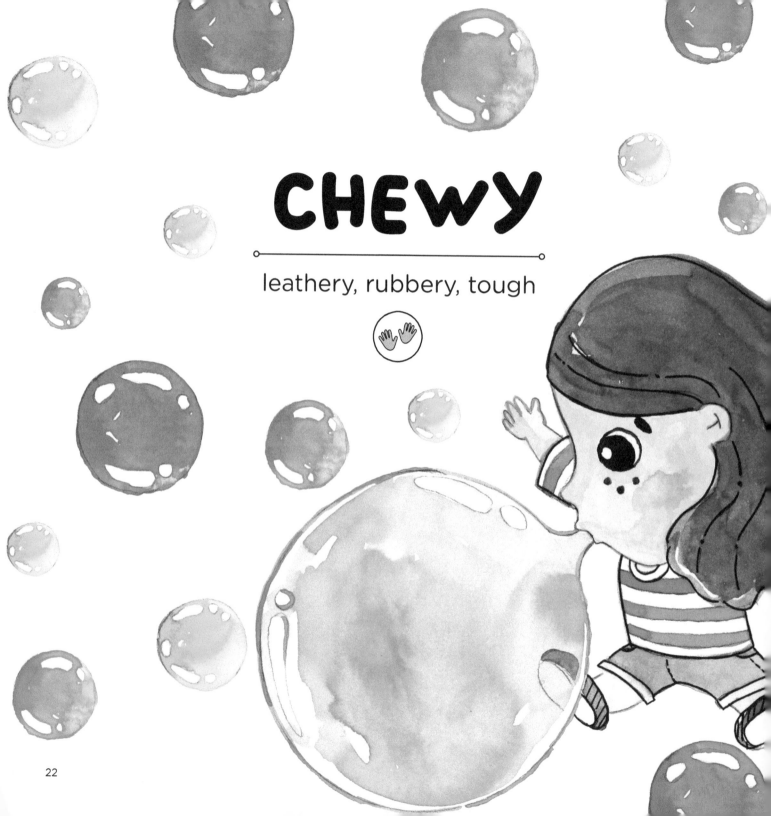

22

CHEWY

leathery, rubbery, tough

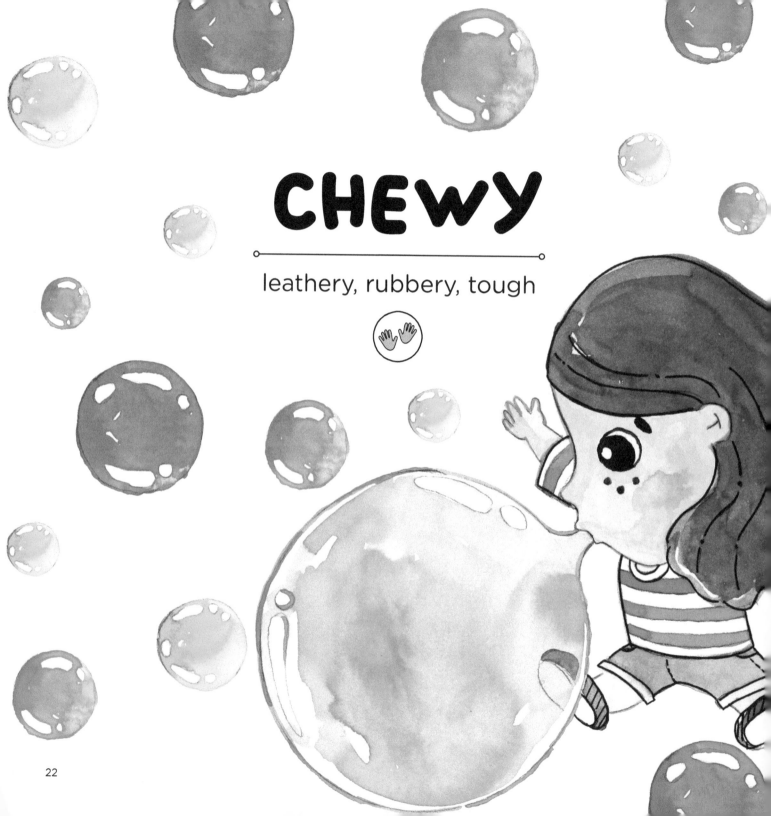

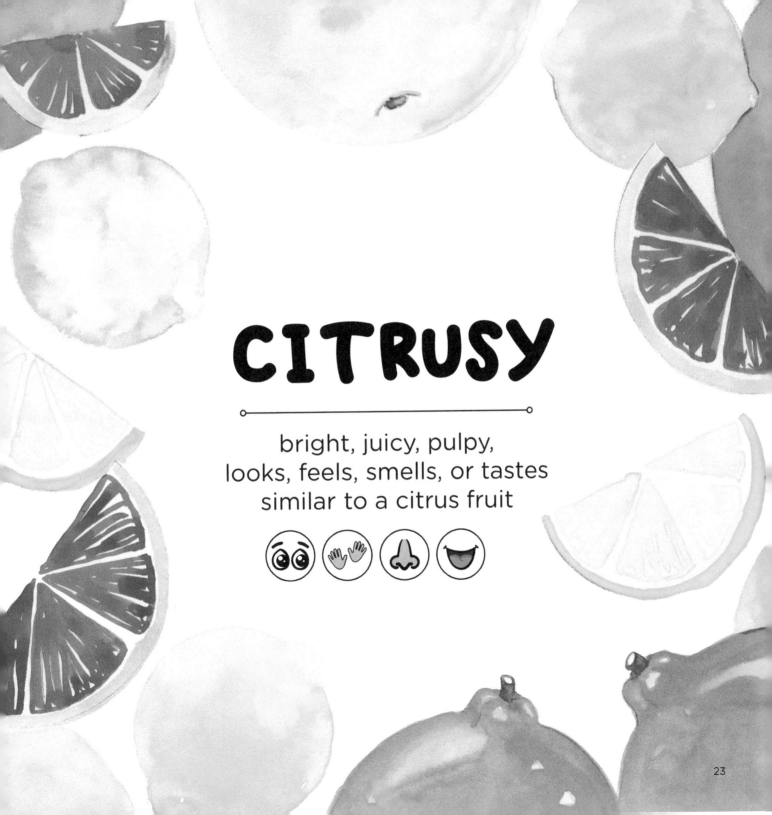

CITRUSY

bright, juicy, pulpy,
looks, feels, smells, or tastes
similar to a citrus fruit

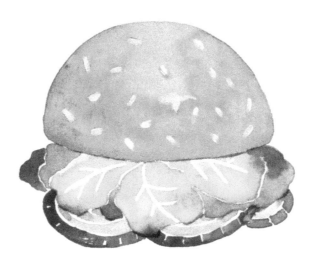

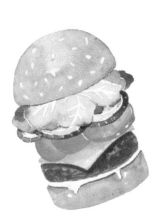

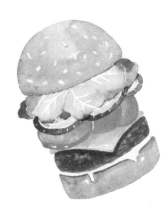

COMPLEX

multiple flavors, textures,
or smells

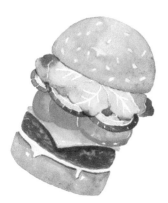

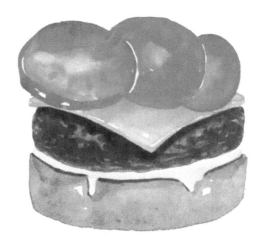

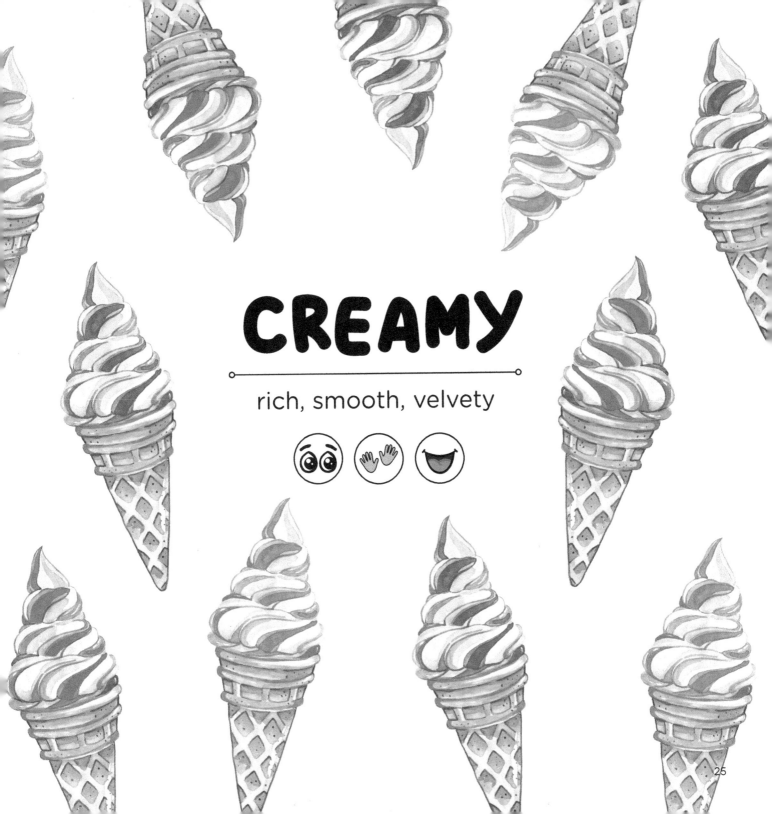

CREAMY

rich, smooth, velvety

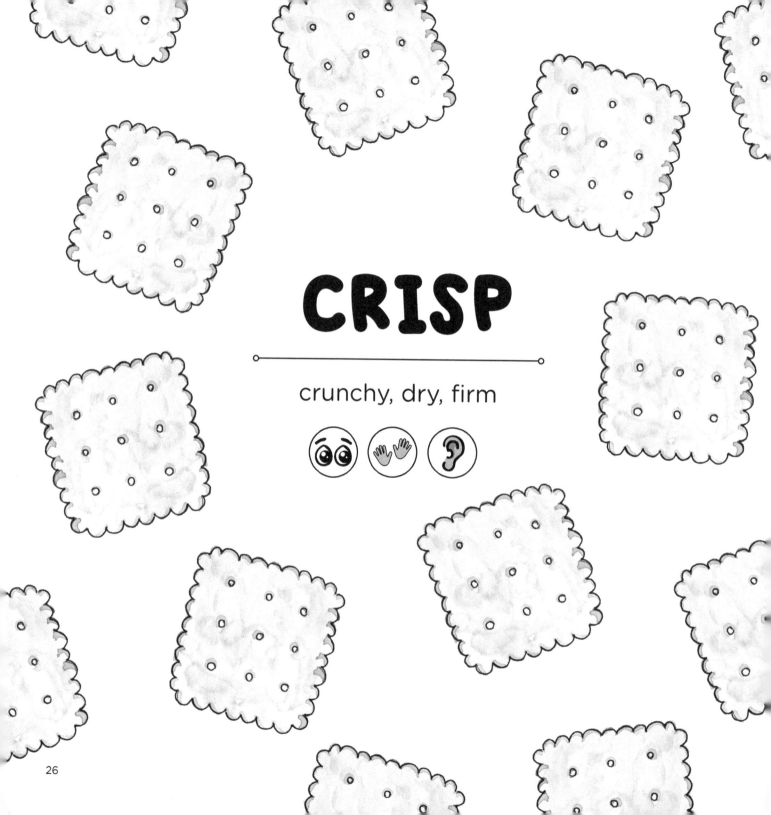

CRISP

crunchy, dry, firm

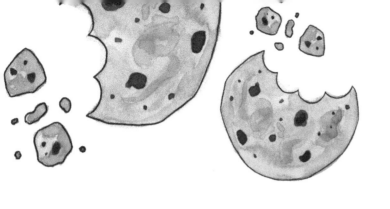
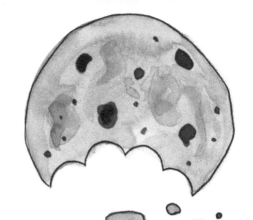

CRUMBLY

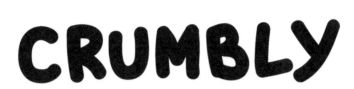

breakable, brittle, crisp

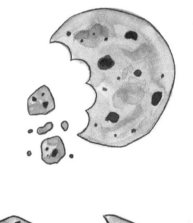
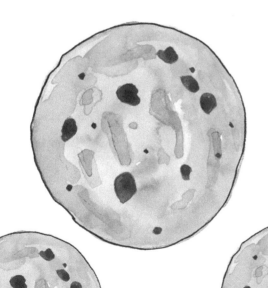
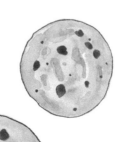
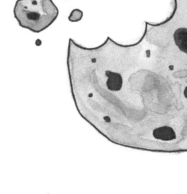

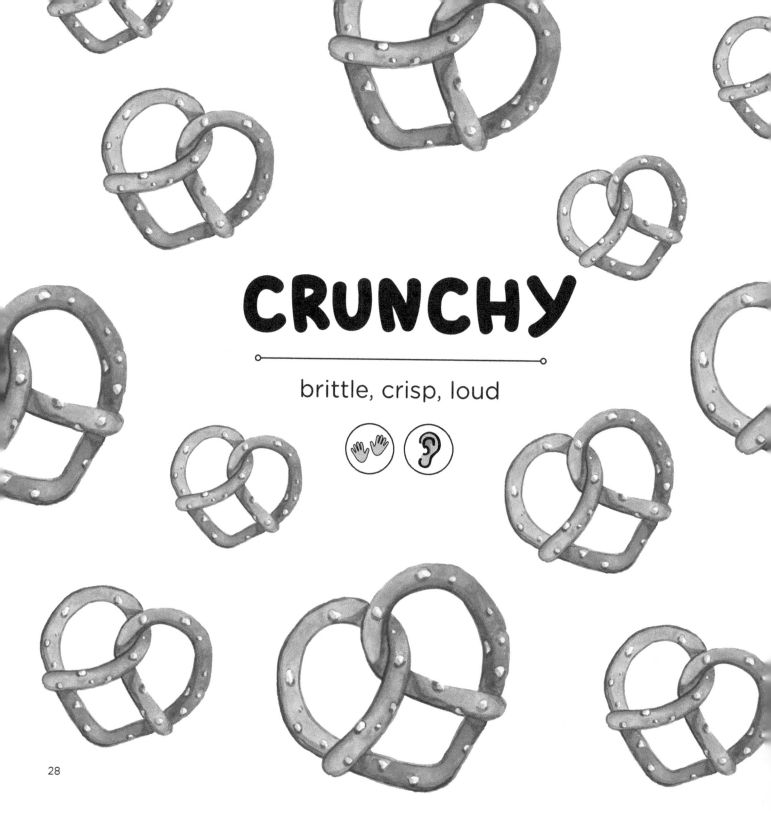

CRUNCHY

brittle, crisp, loud

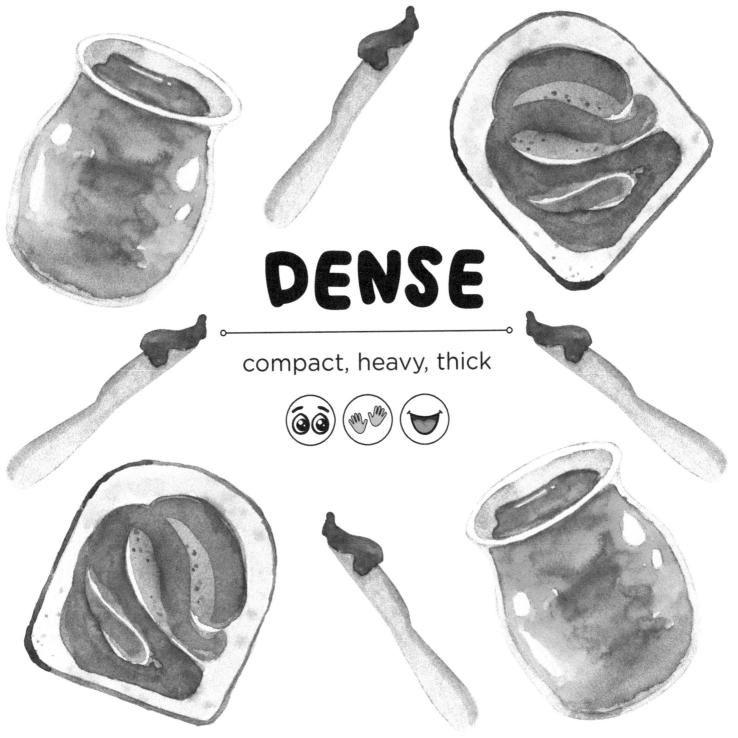

DENSE

compact, heavy, thick

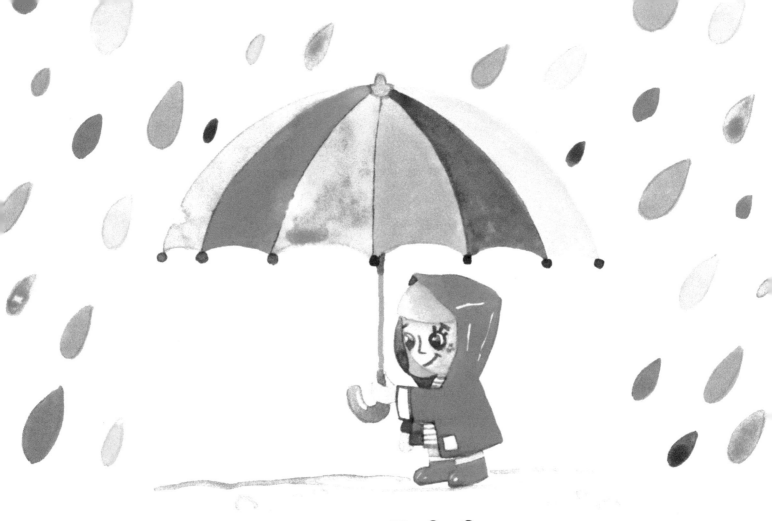

DRY

having no or very little
water or moisture

DULL

bland, boring, unexciting

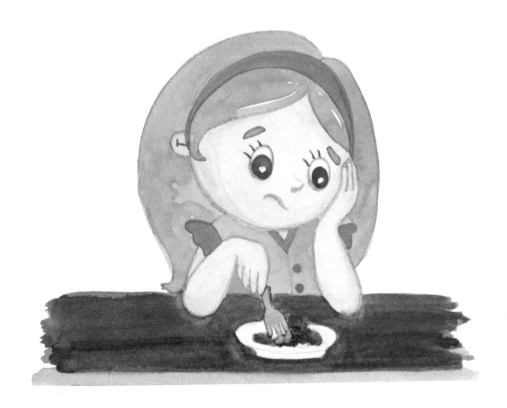

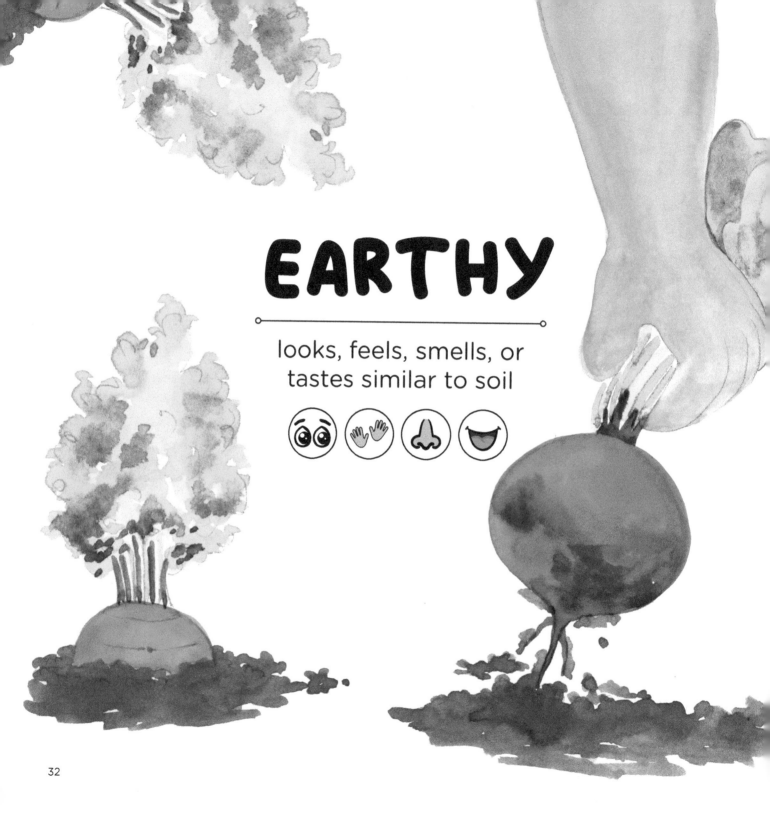

EARTHY

looks, feels, smells, or
tastes similar to soil

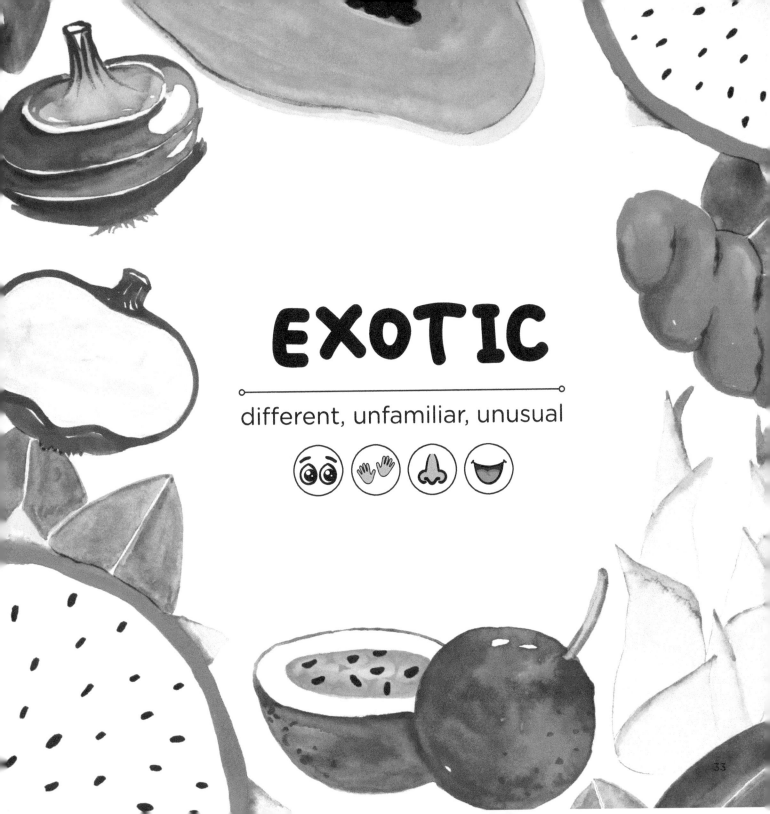

EXOTIC

different, unfamiliar, unusual

33

FIBROUS

stringy, thick, tough

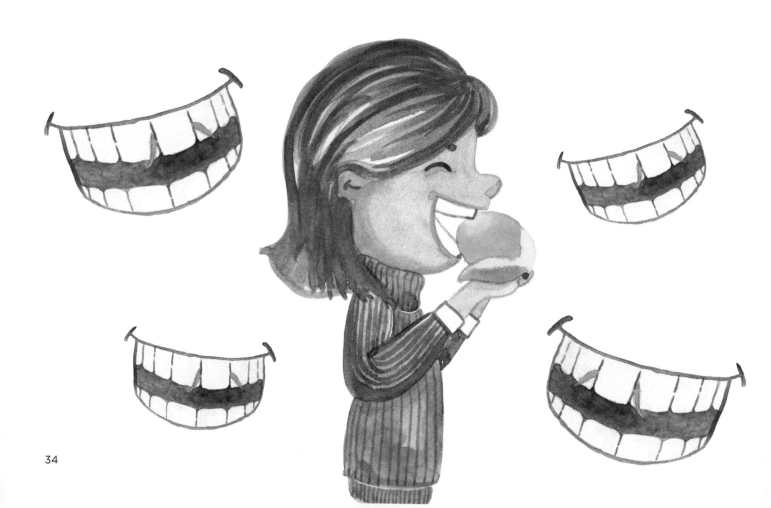

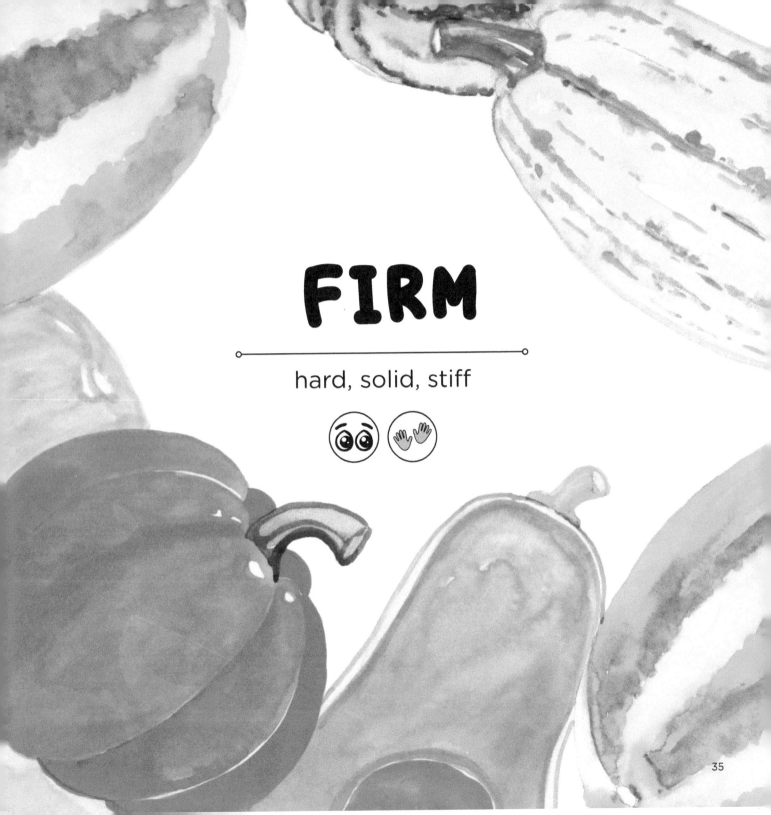

FIRM

hard, solid, stiff

FLAVORFUL

having a lot of flavor

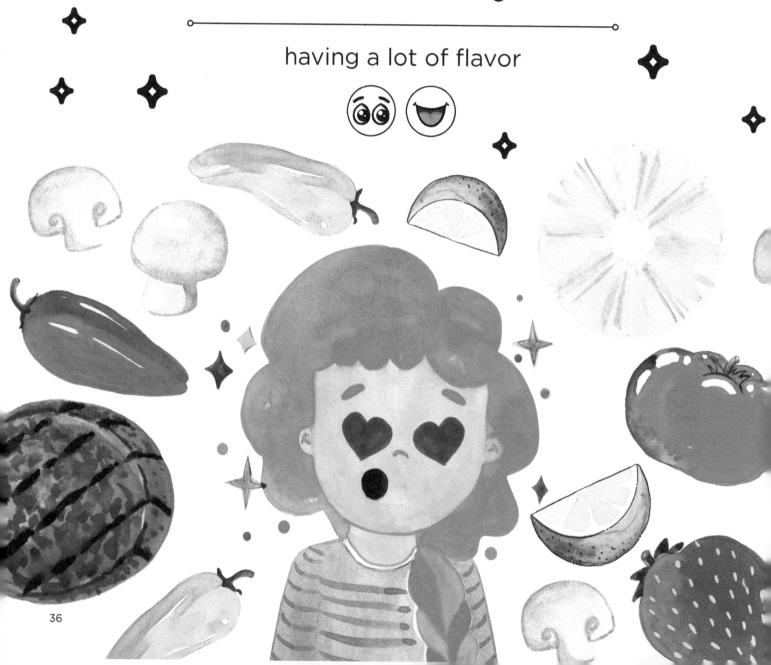

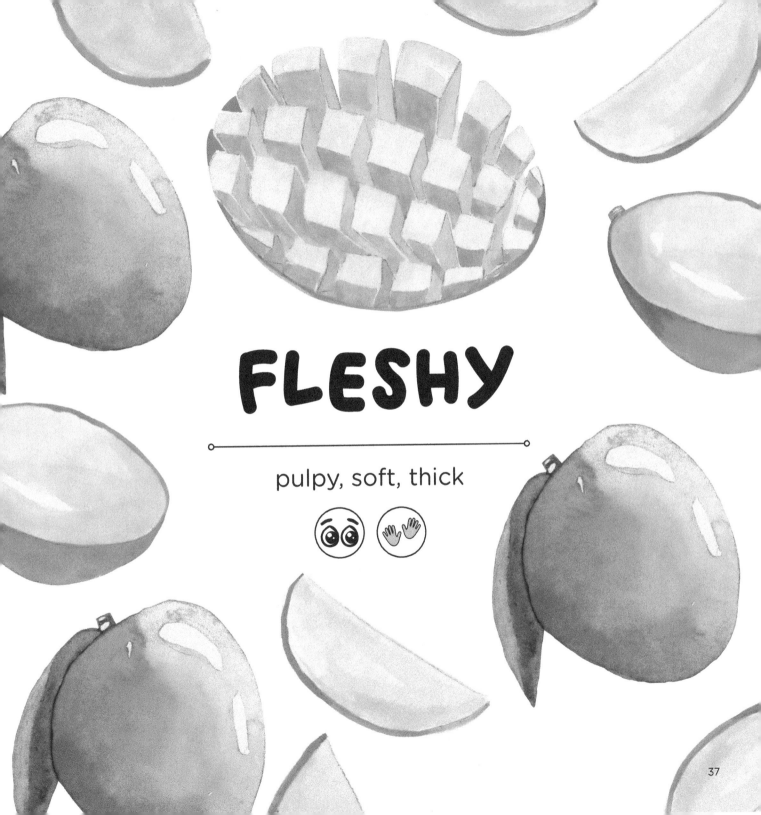

FLESHY

pulpy, soft, thick

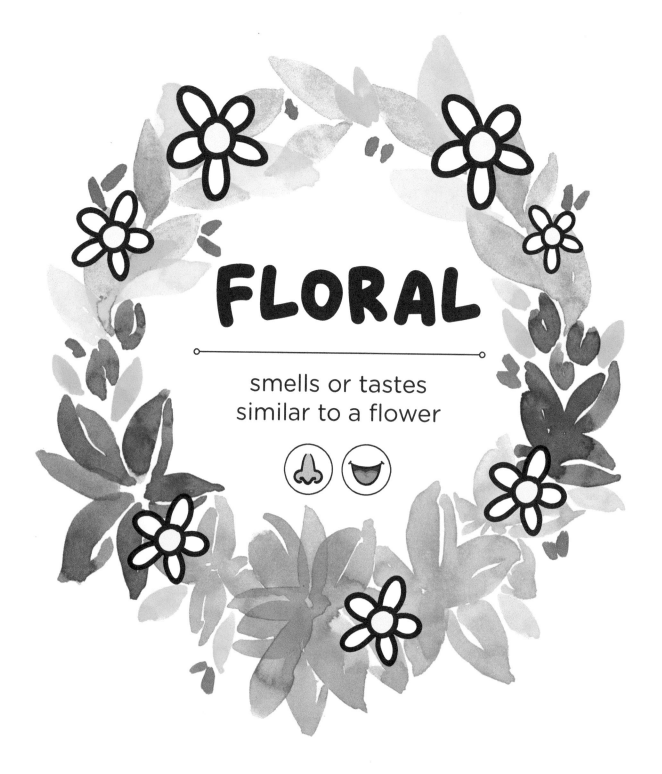

FLORAL

smells or tastes
similar to a flower

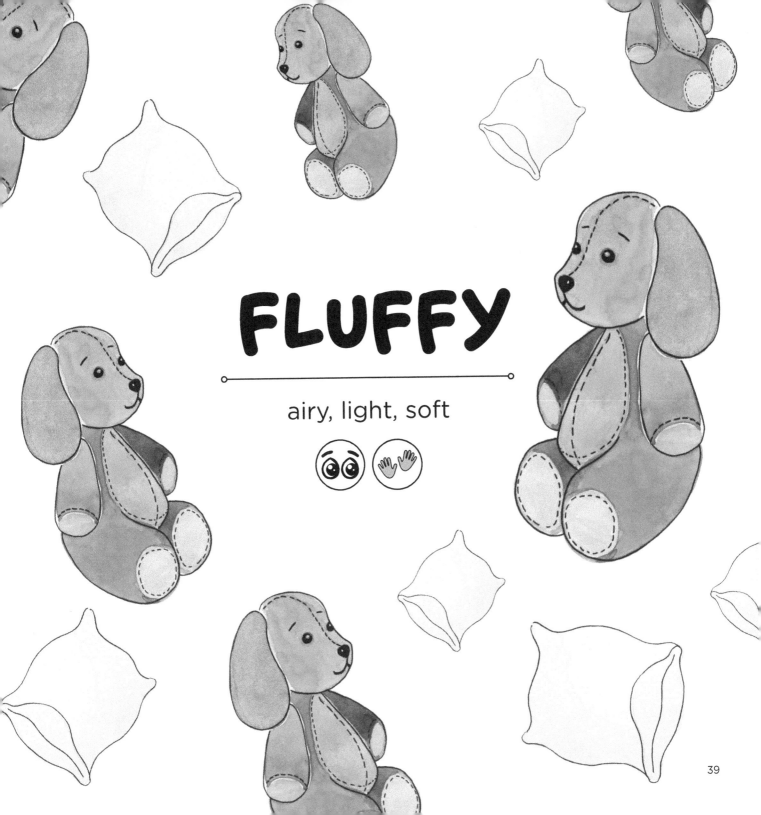

FLUFFY

airy, light, soft

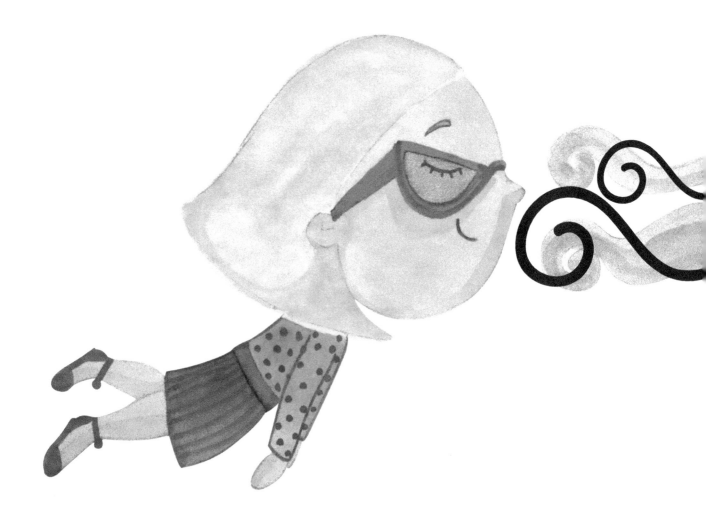

FRAGRANT

nice or sweet smell, perfumed

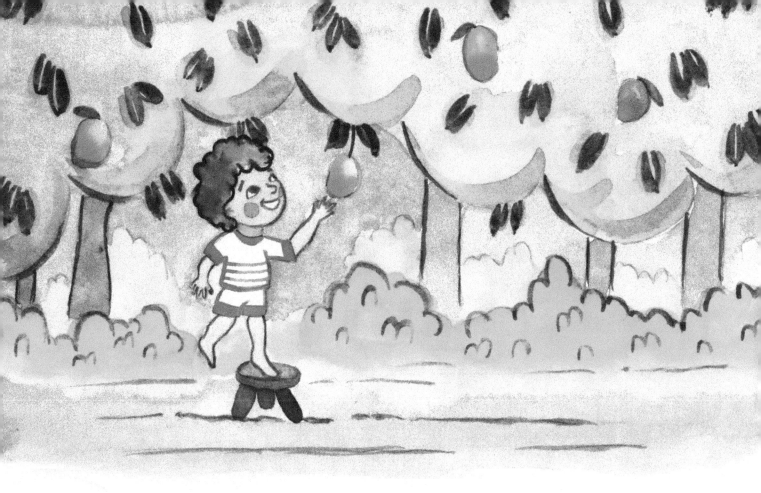

FRESH

new, ripe, unspoiled

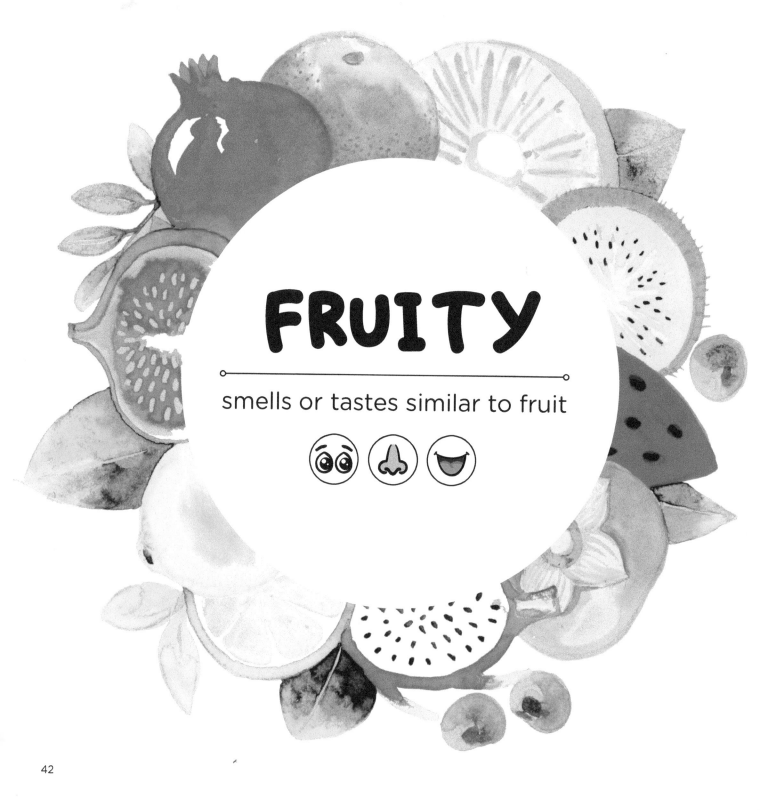

FRUITY

smells or tastes similar to fruit

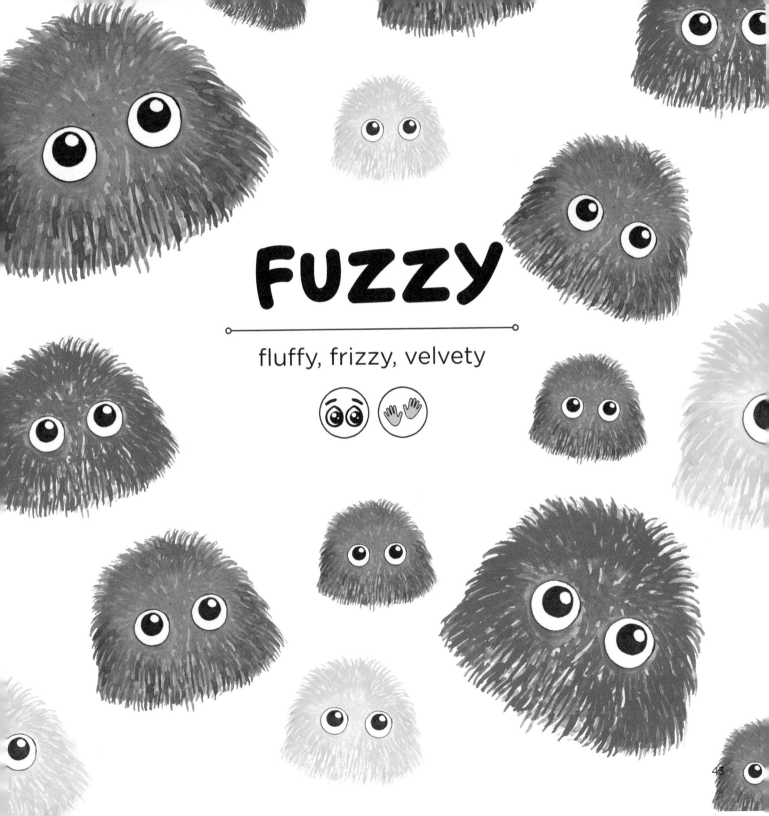

FUZZY

fluffy, frizzy, velvety

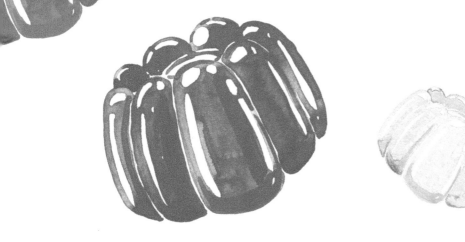
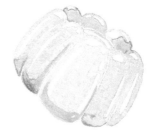
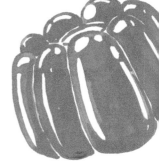

GELATINOUS

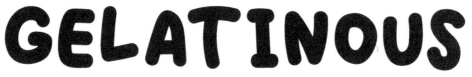

gluey, jelly-like, sticky

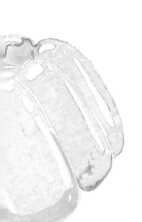
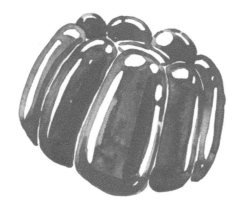
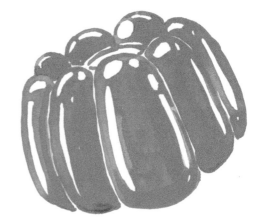

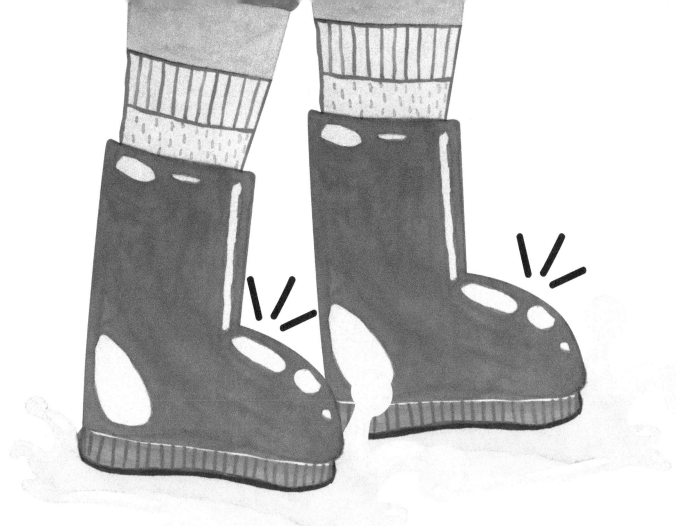

GLOSSY

glazed, polished, shiny

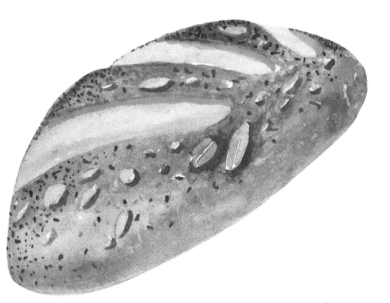

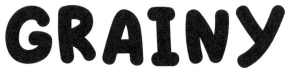

GRAINY

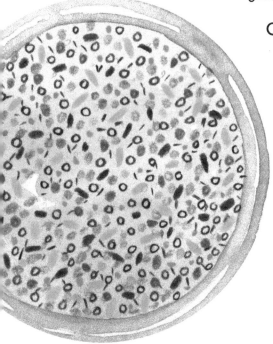

coarse, granular, gritty

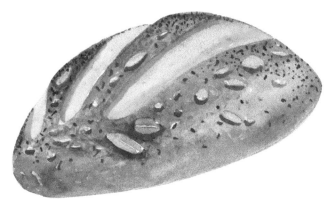

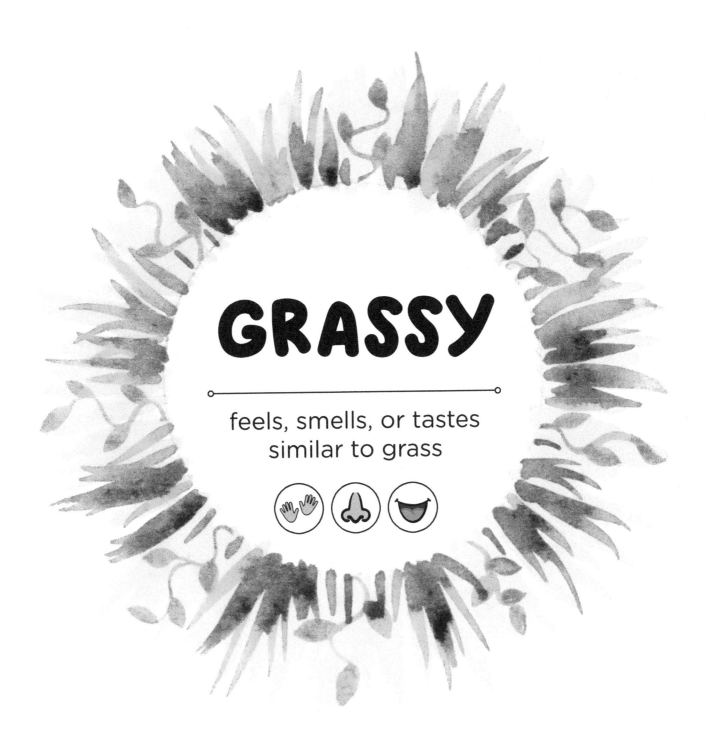

GRASSY

feels, smells, or tastes
similar to grass

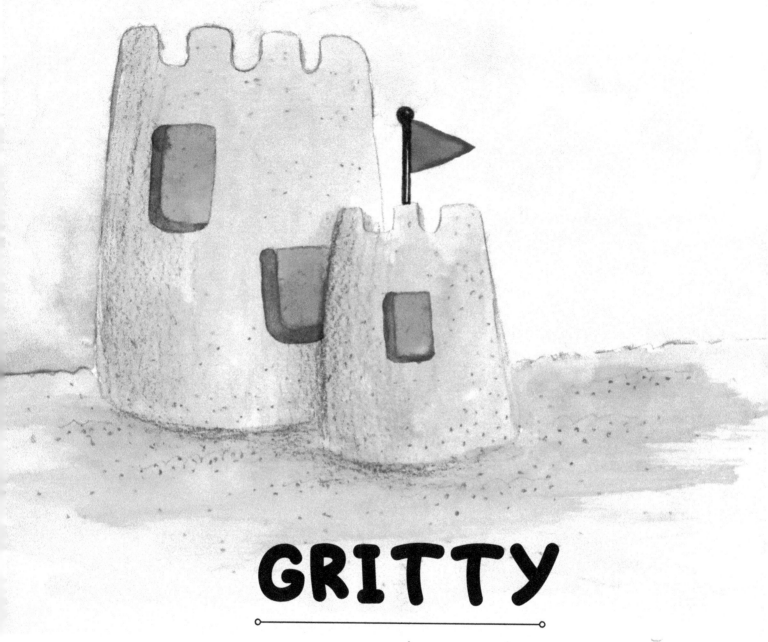

GRITTY

coarse, grainy, rough

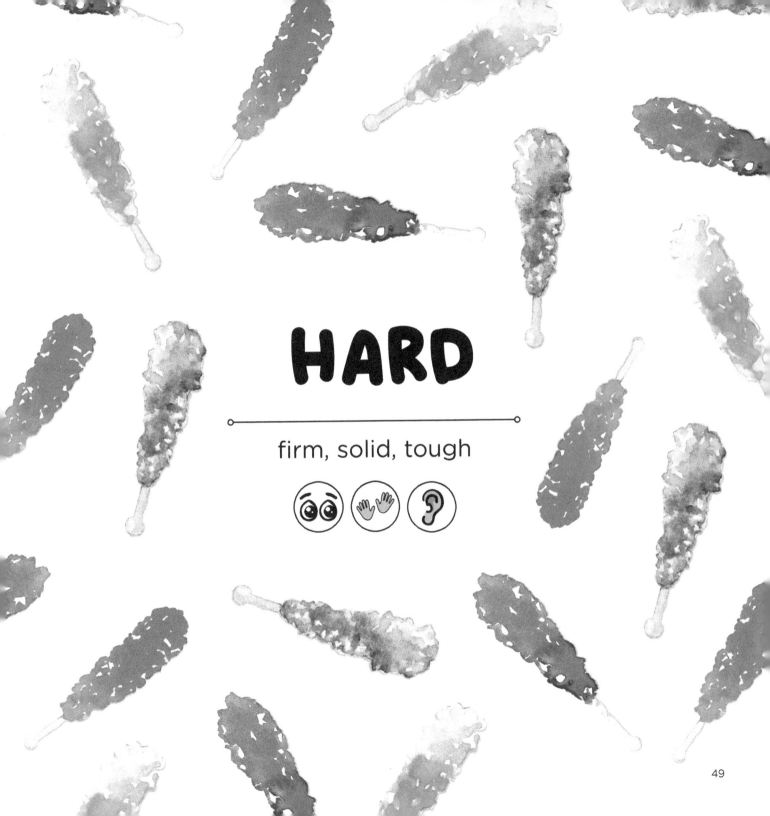

HARD

firm, solid, tough

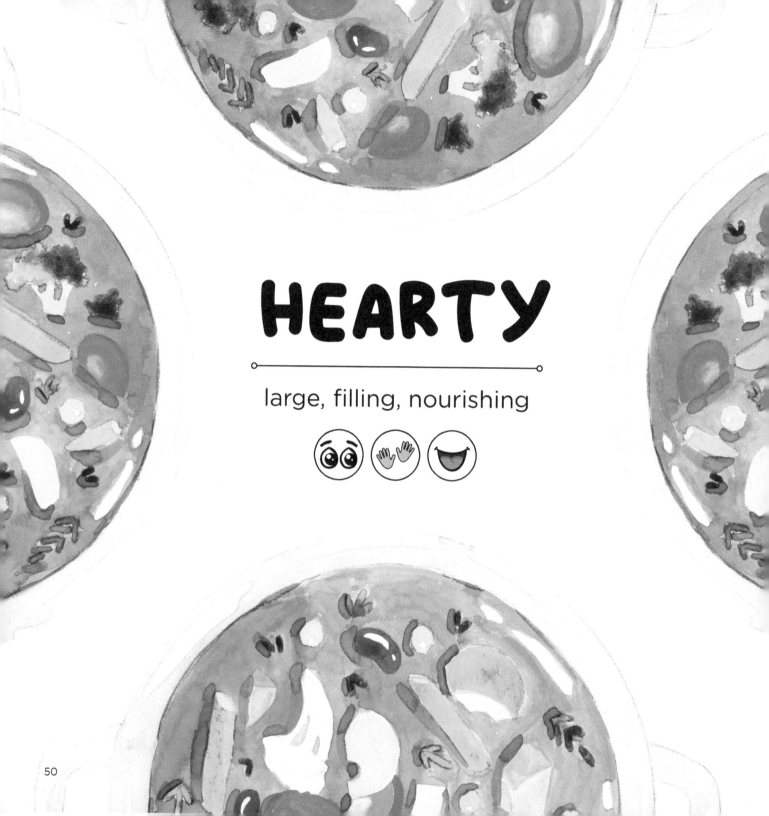

HEARTY

large, filling, nourishing

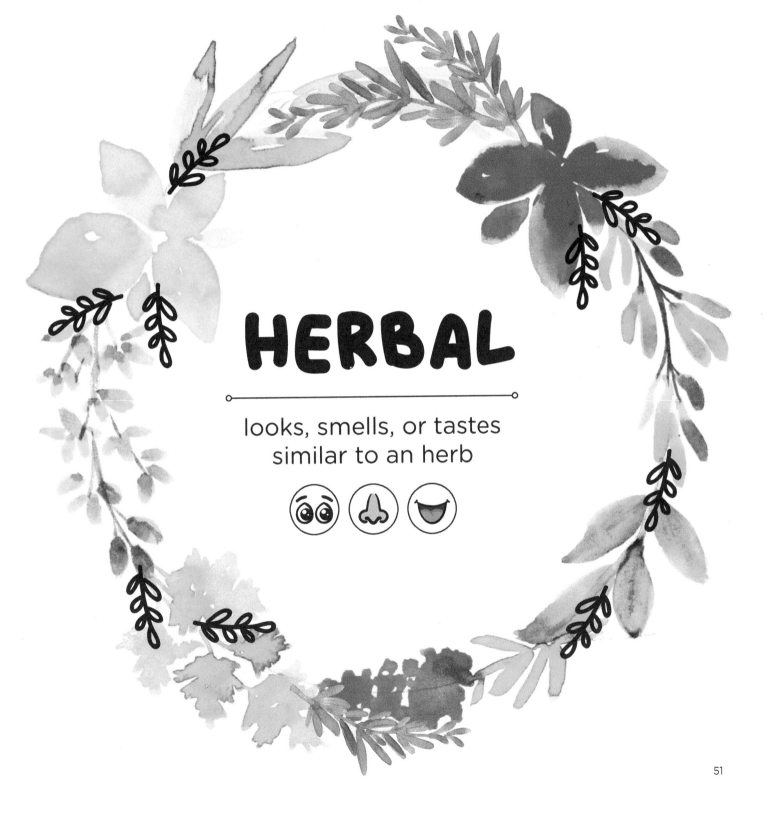

HERBAL

looks, smells, or tastes
similar to an herb

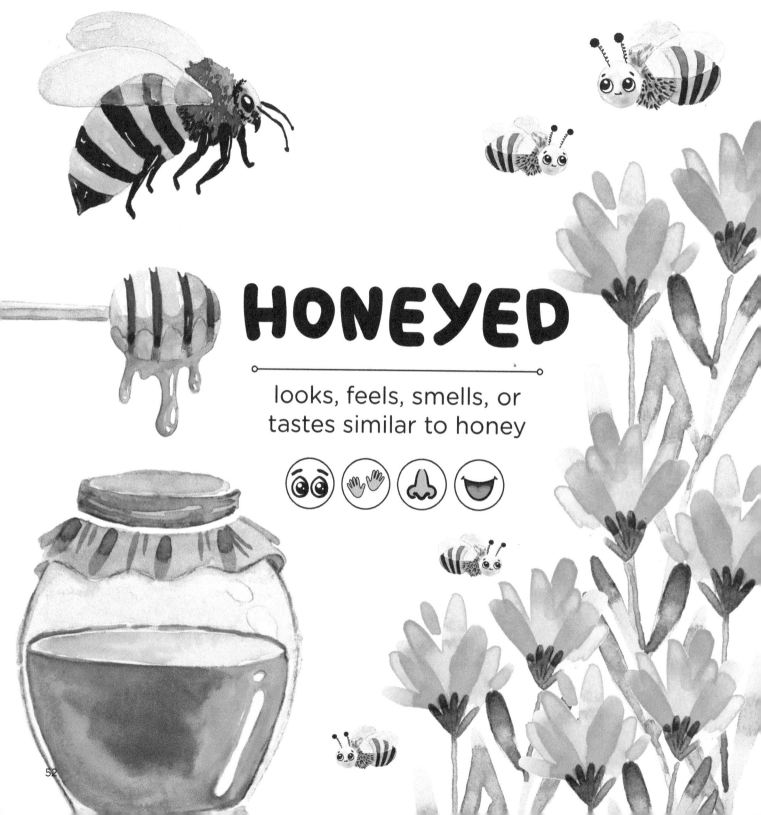

HONEYED

looks, feels, smells, or
tastes similar to honey

52

INTENSE

sharp, strong, powerful

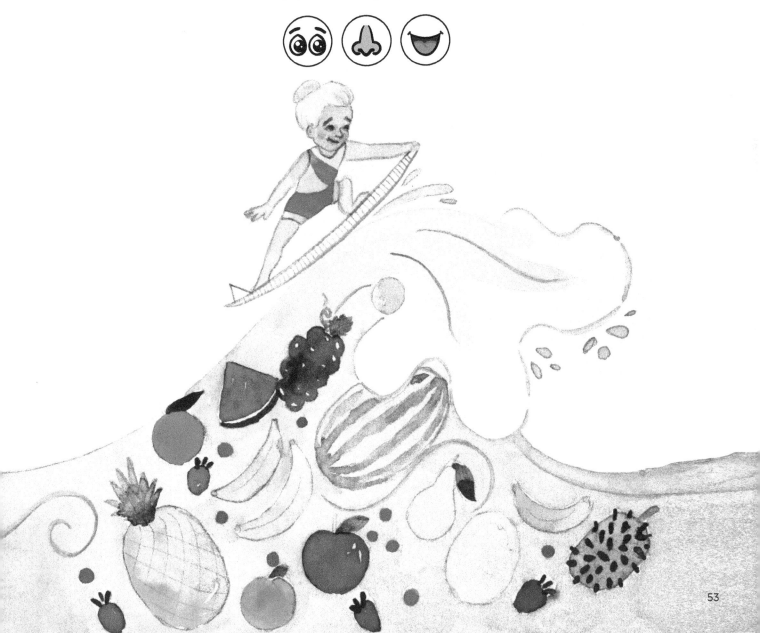

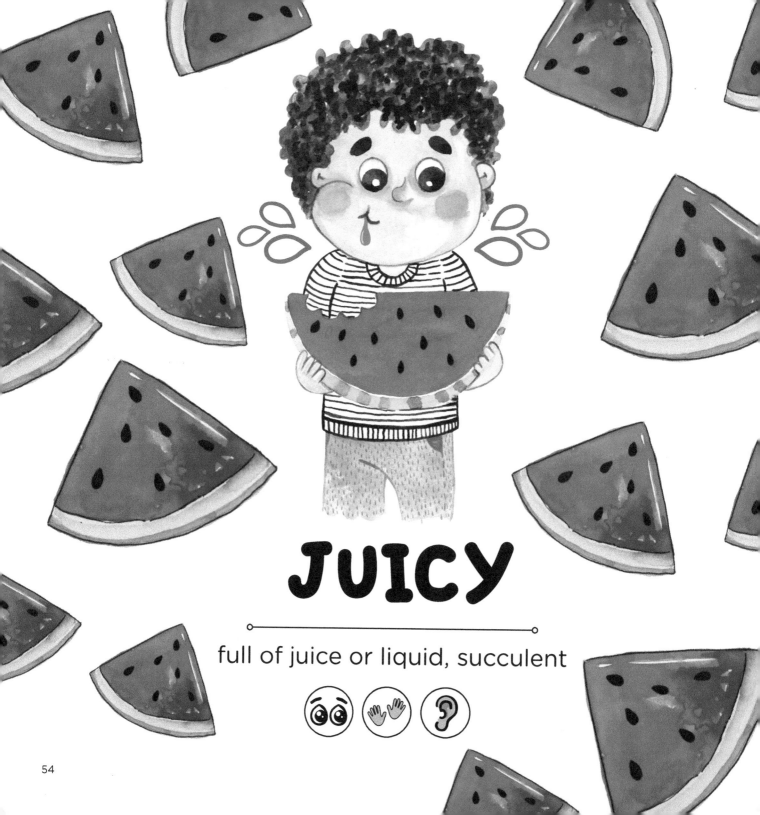

JUICY

full of juice or liquid, succulent

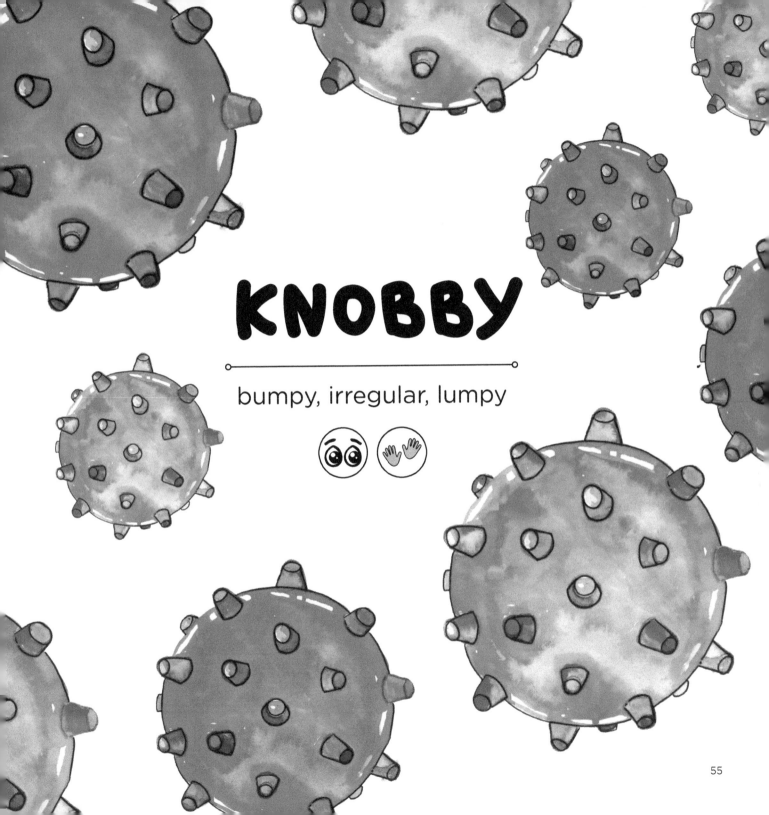

KNOBBY

bumpy, irregular, lumpy

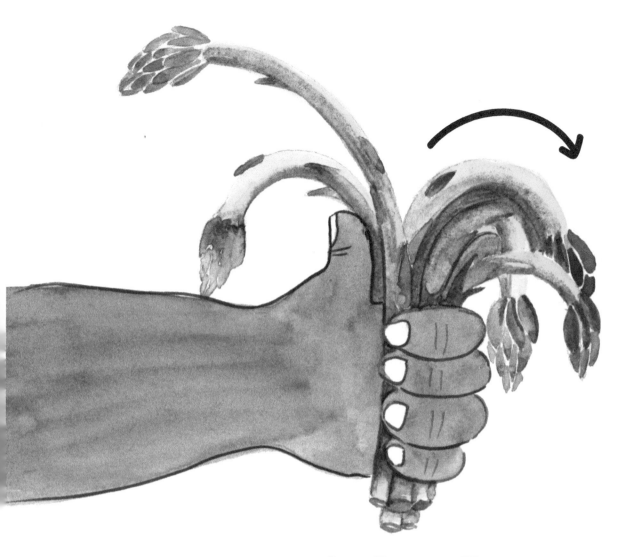

LIMP

floppy, lifeless, soft

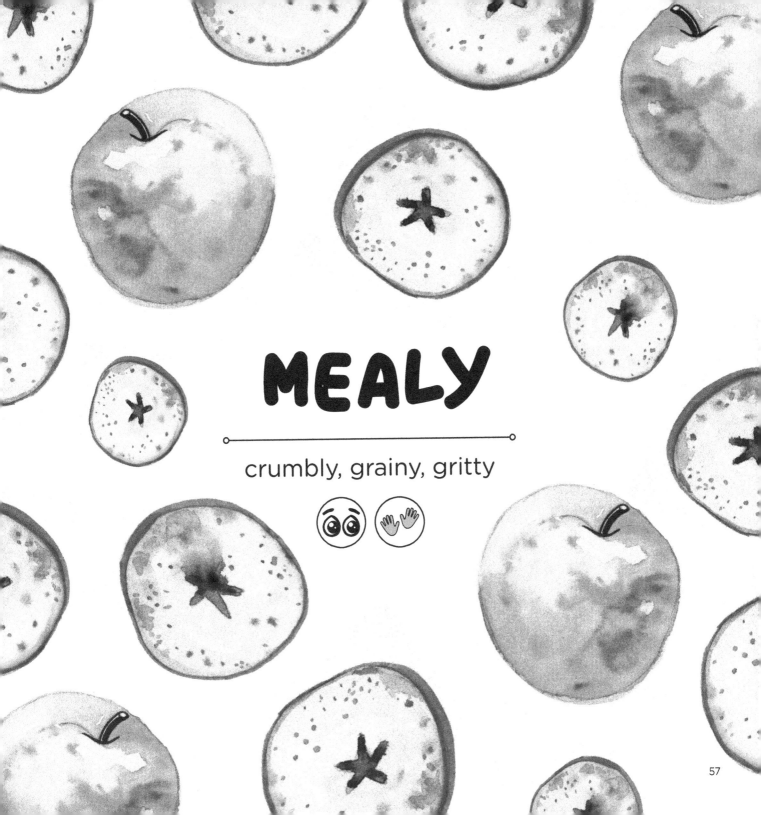

MEALY

crumbly, grainy, gritty

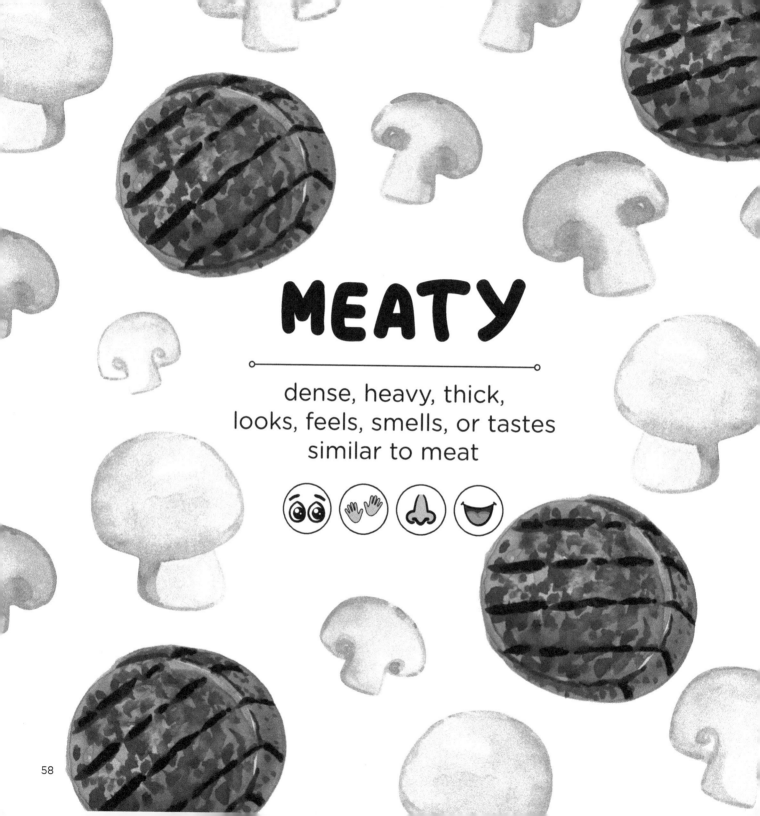

MEATY

dense, heavy, thick,
looks, feels, smells, or tastes
similar to meat

MELTY

dissolve, liquify, soften

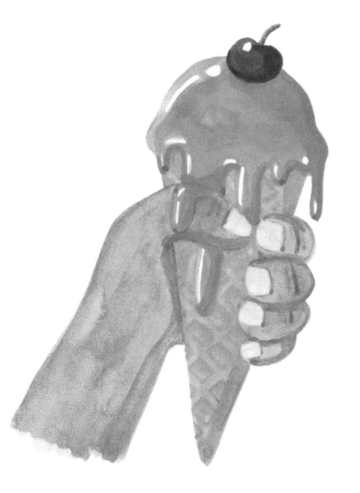 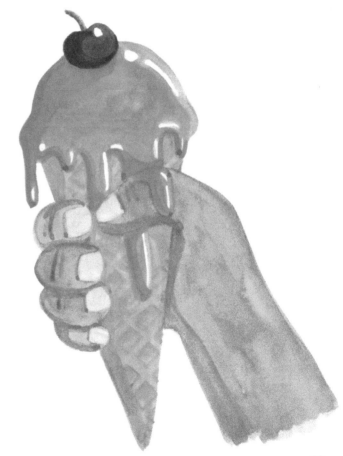

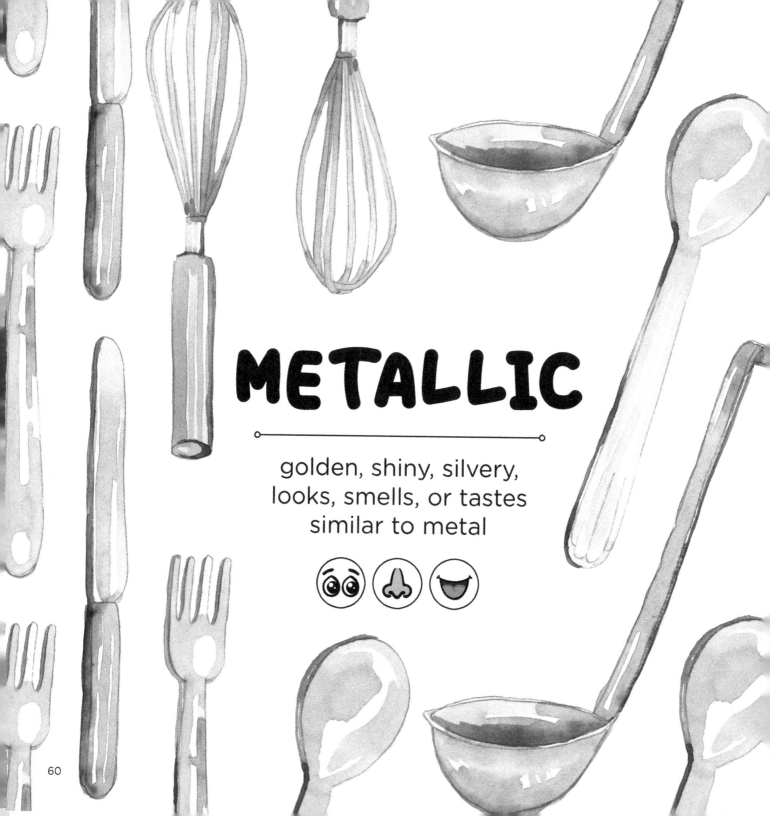

METALLIC

golden, shiny, silvery,
looks, smells, or tastes
similar to metal

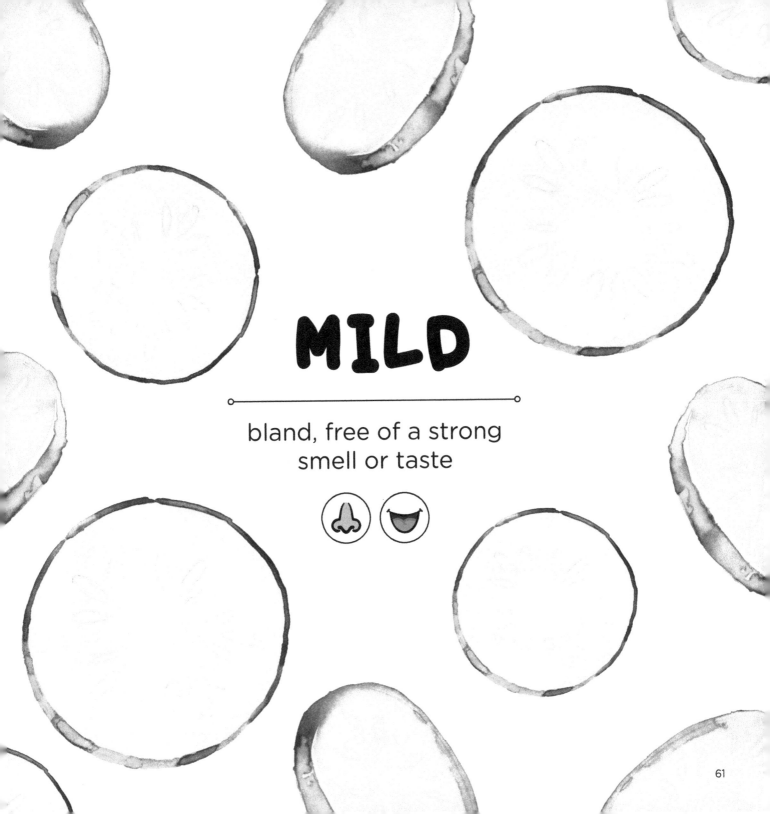

MILD

bland, free of a strong
smell or taste

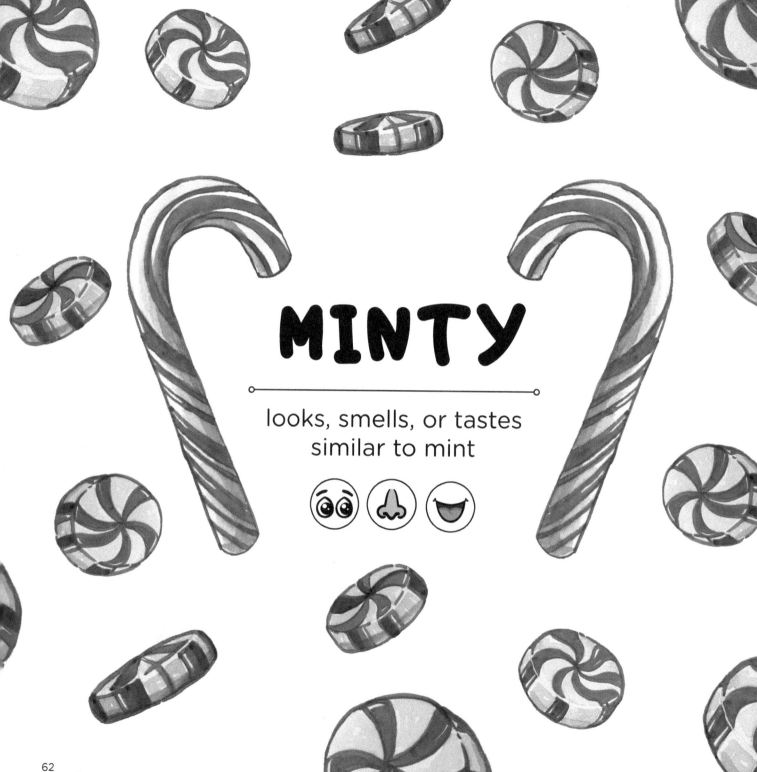

MINTY

looks, smells, or tastes
similar to mint

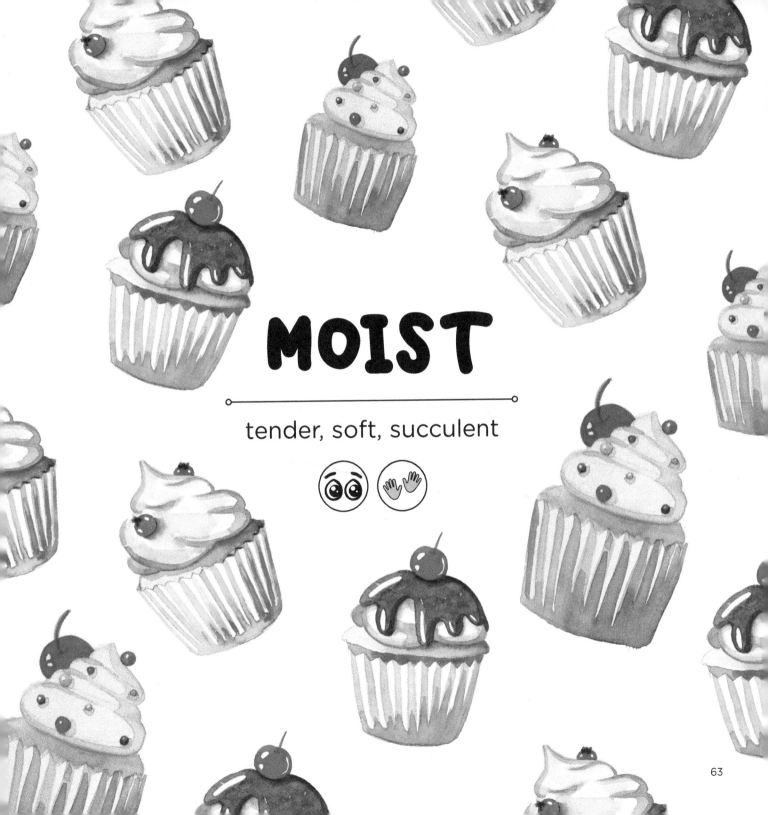

MOIST

tender, soft, succulent

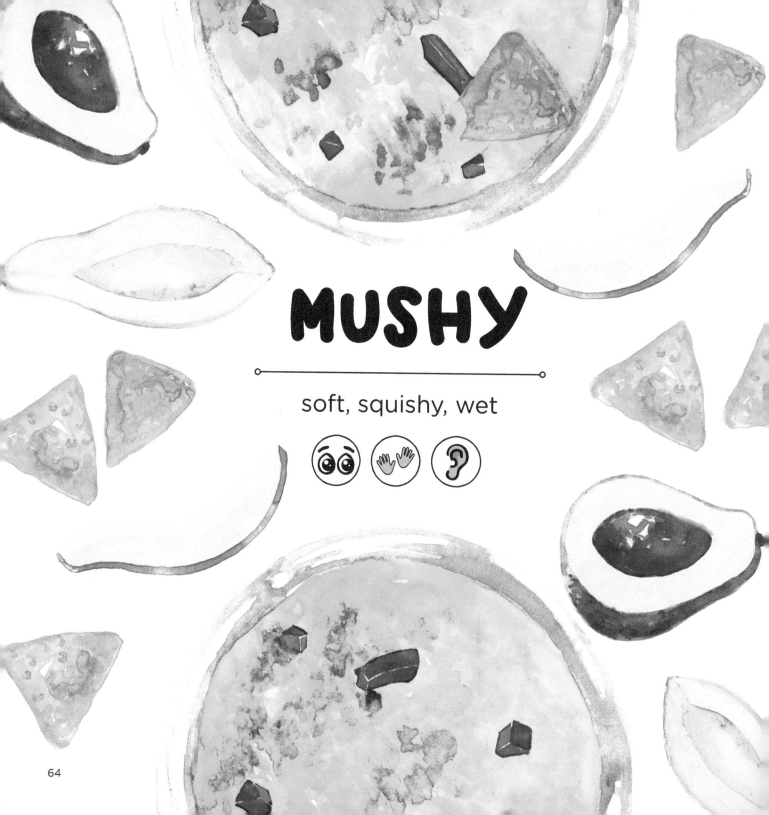

MUSHY

soft, squishy, wet

MUSKY

strong, natural scent, piquant

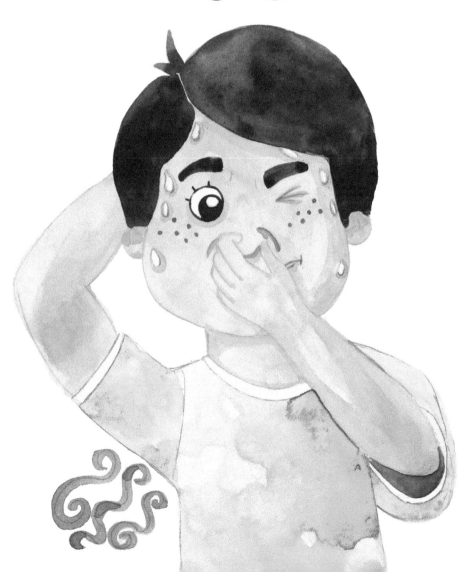

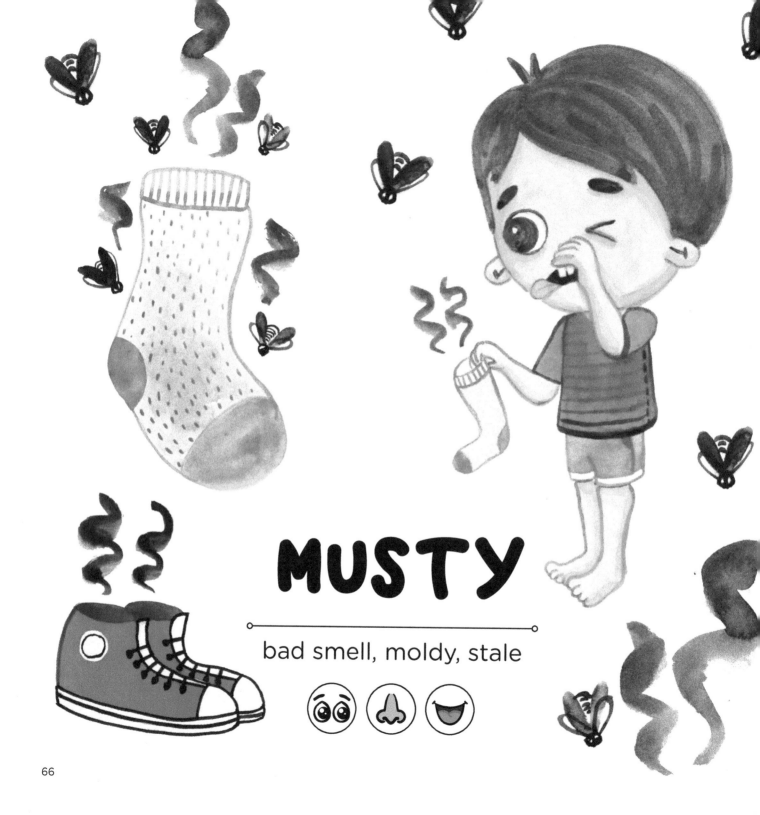

MUSTY

bad smell, moldy, stale

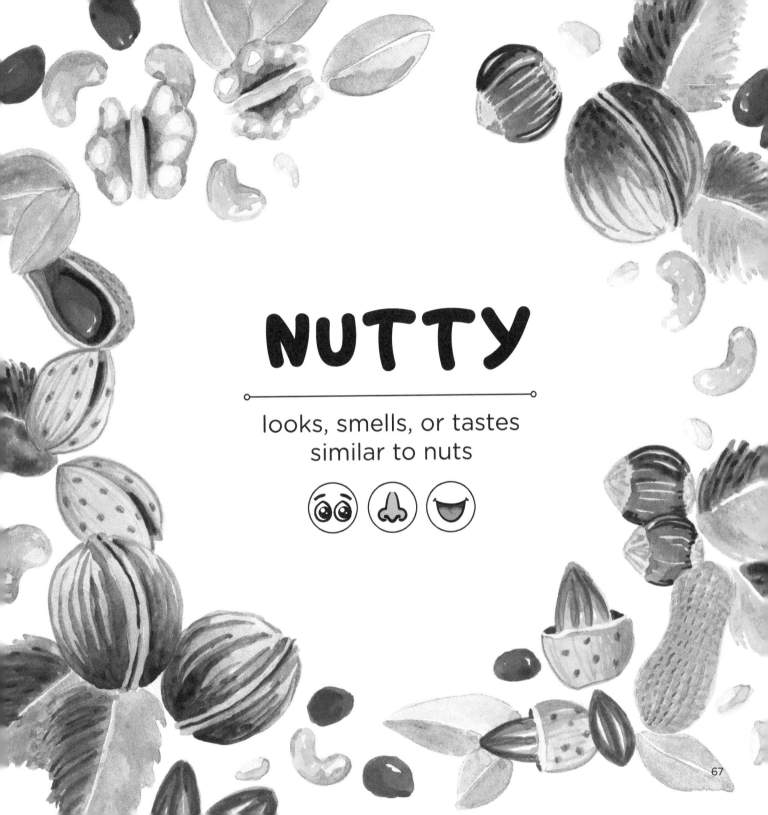

NUTTY

looks, smells, or tastes
similar to nuts

ODOR

aroma, scent, smell

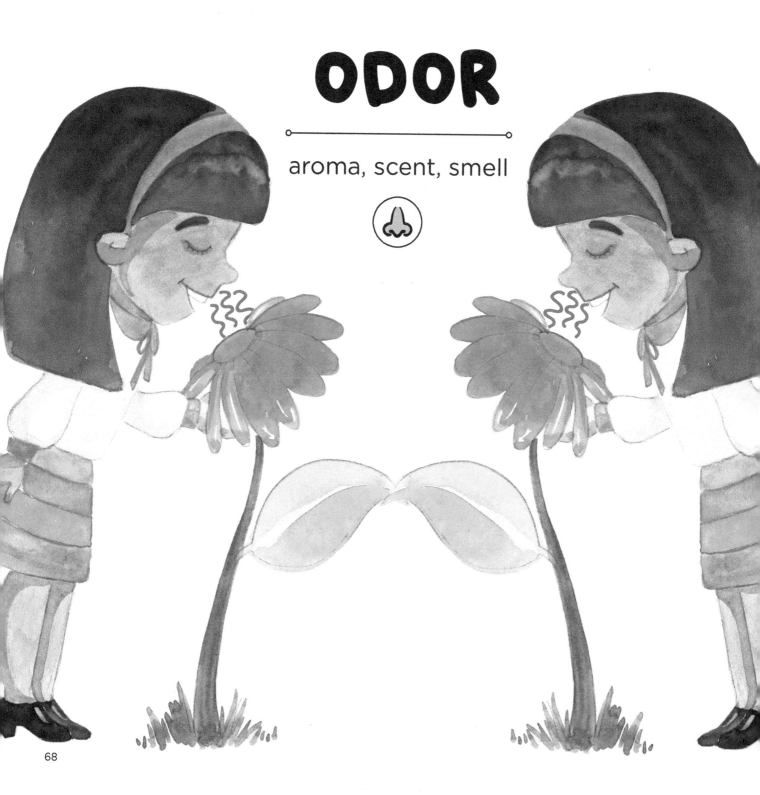

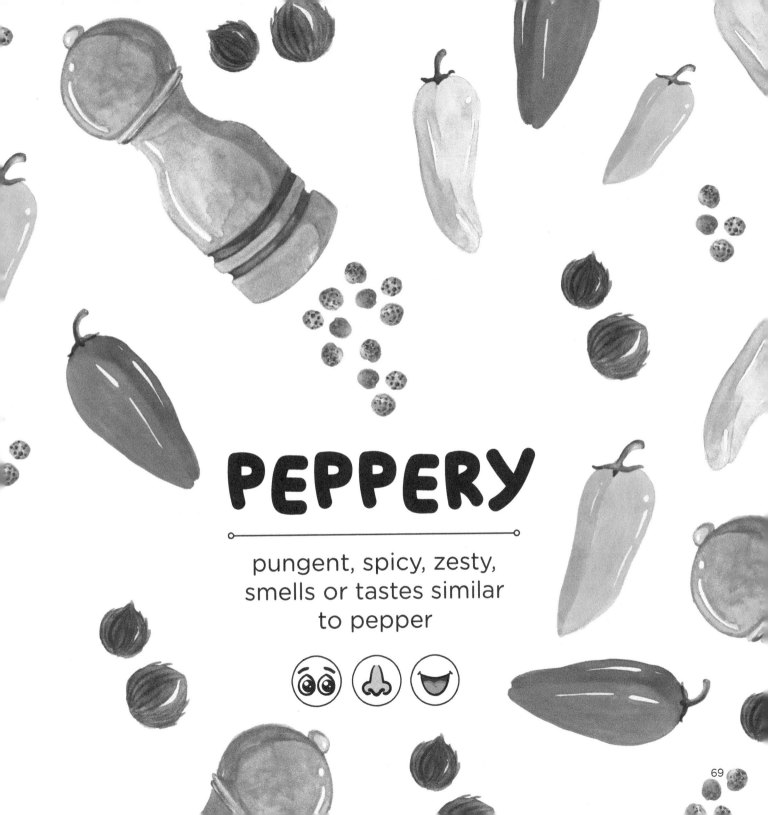

PEPPERY

pungent, spicy, zesty,
smells or tastes similar
to pepper

PIQUANT

flavorful, tangy, zesty

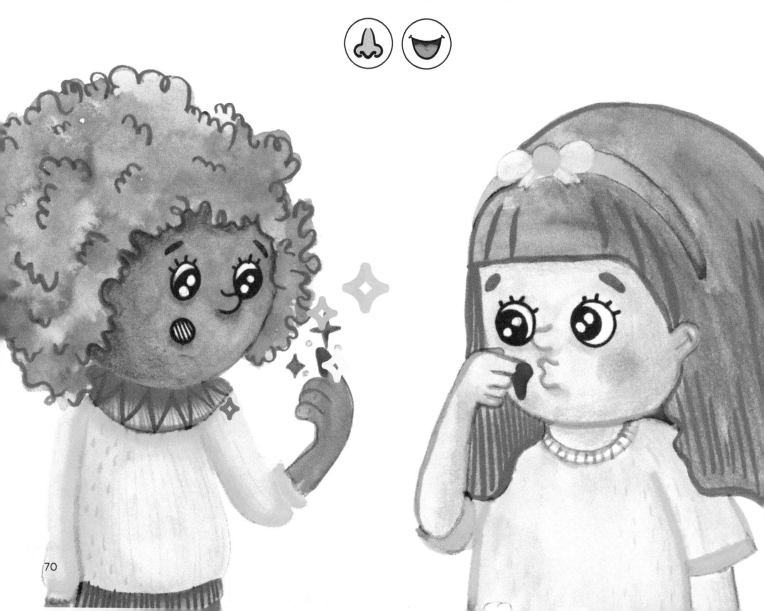

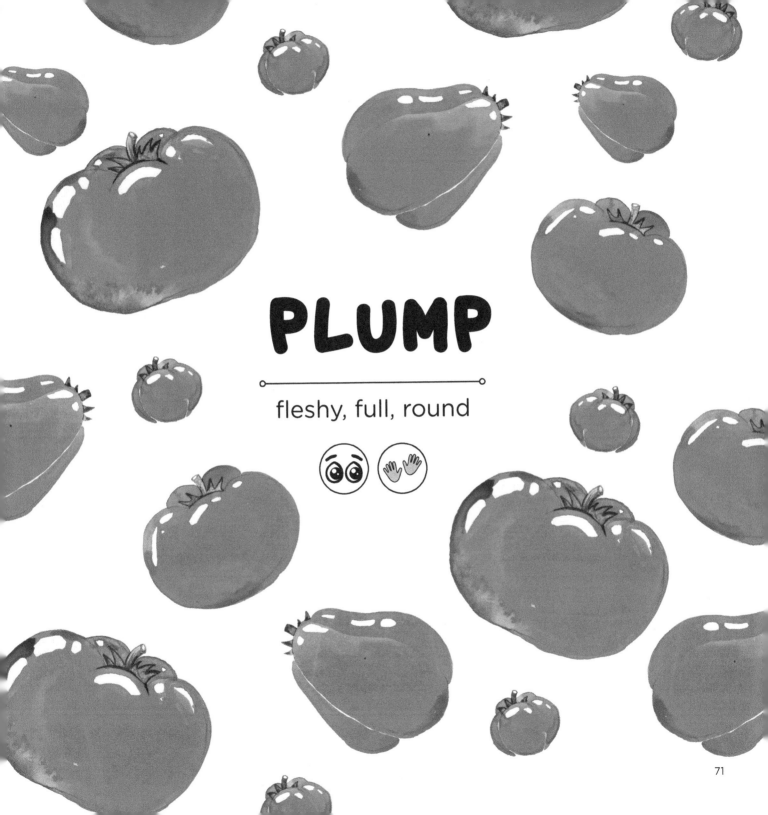

PLUMP

fleshy, full, round

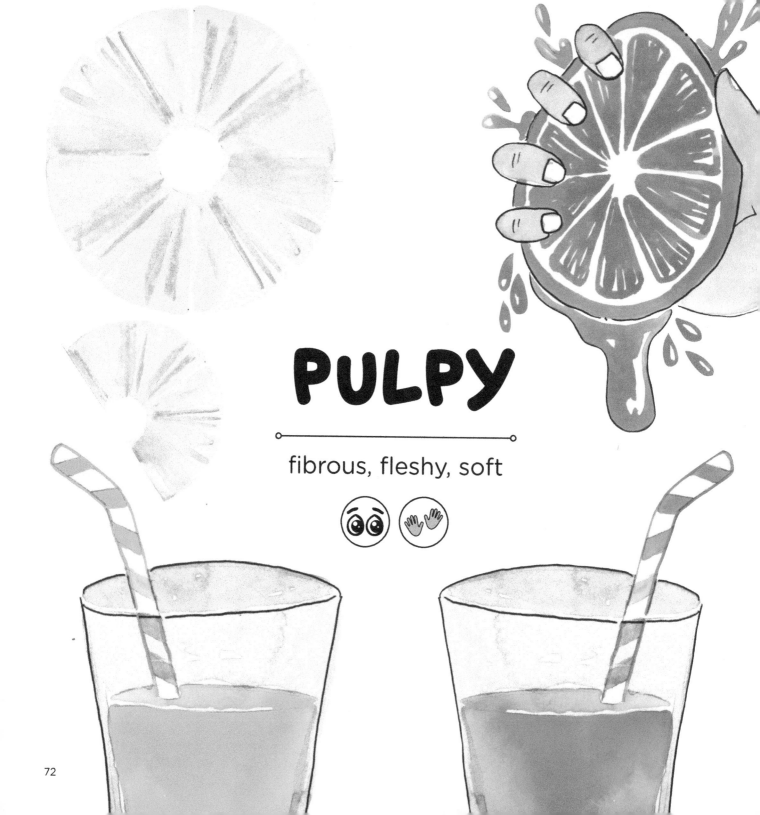

PULPY

fibrous, fleshy, soft

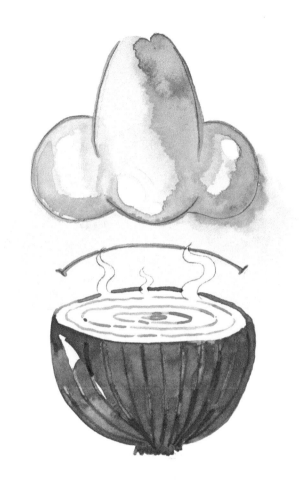

PUNGENT

aromatic, piquant, sharp,
strong smell or taste

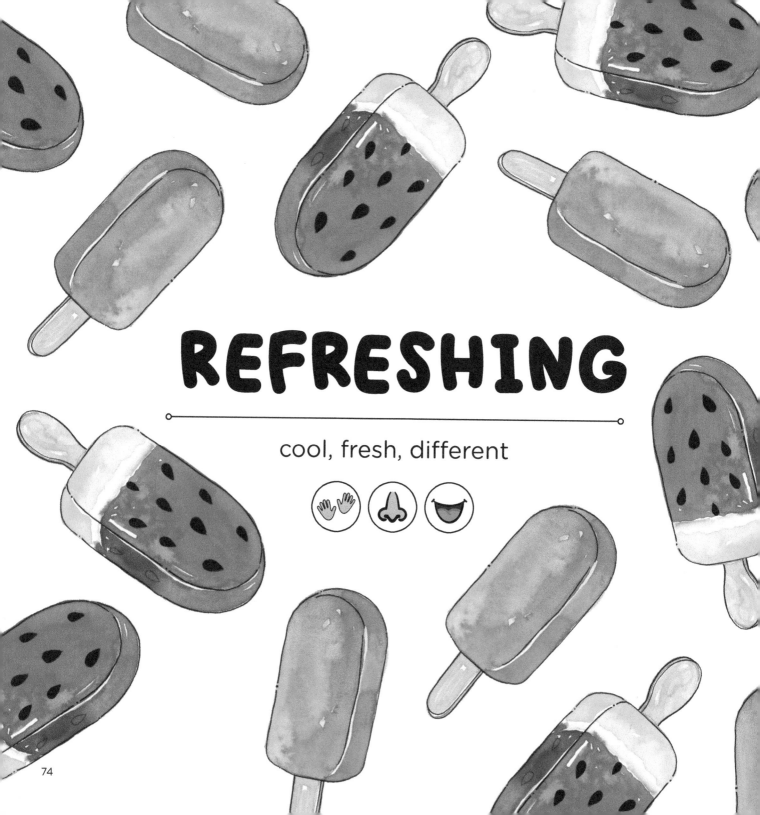

REFRESHING

cool, fresh, different

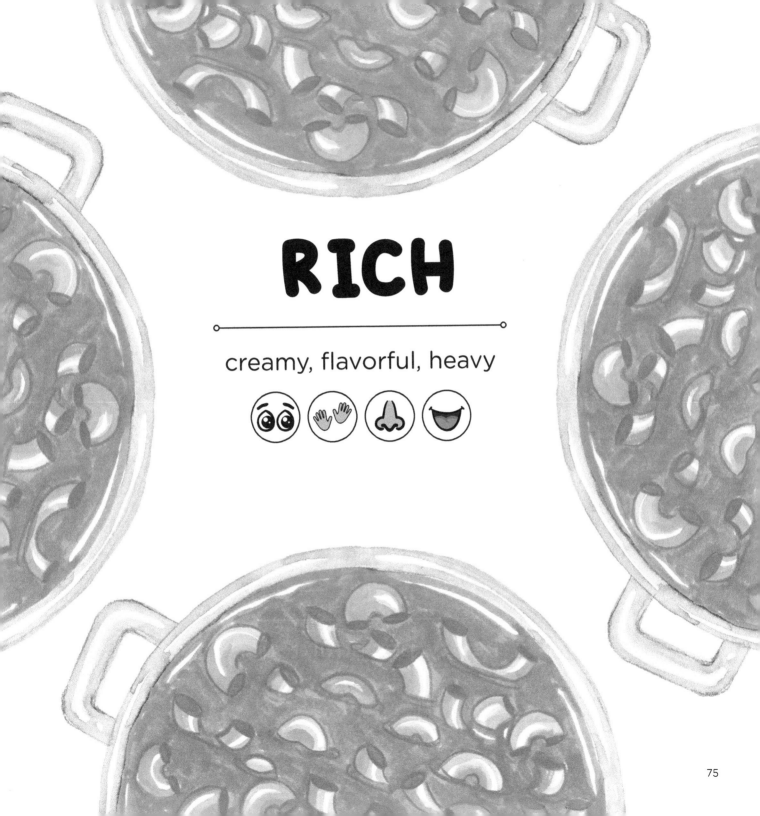

RICH

creamy, flavorful, heavy

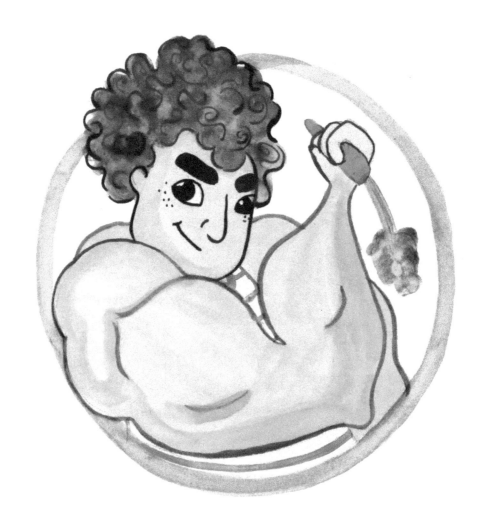

ROBUST

hearty, powerful, tough

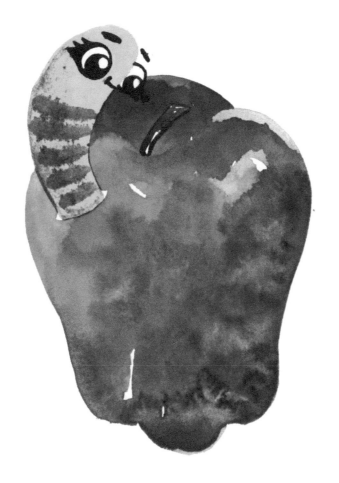

ROTTEN

moldy, over-ripe, spoiled

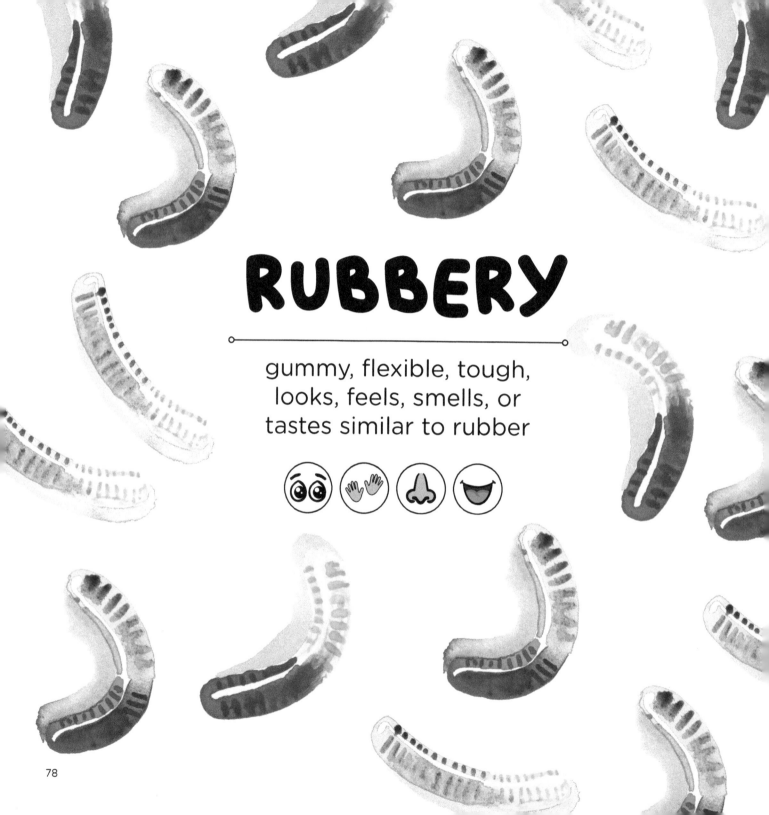

RUBBERY

gummy, flexible, tough, looks, feels, smells, or tastes similar to rubber

SALTY

briny, flavorsome, piquant,
looks, feels, or tastes
similar to salt

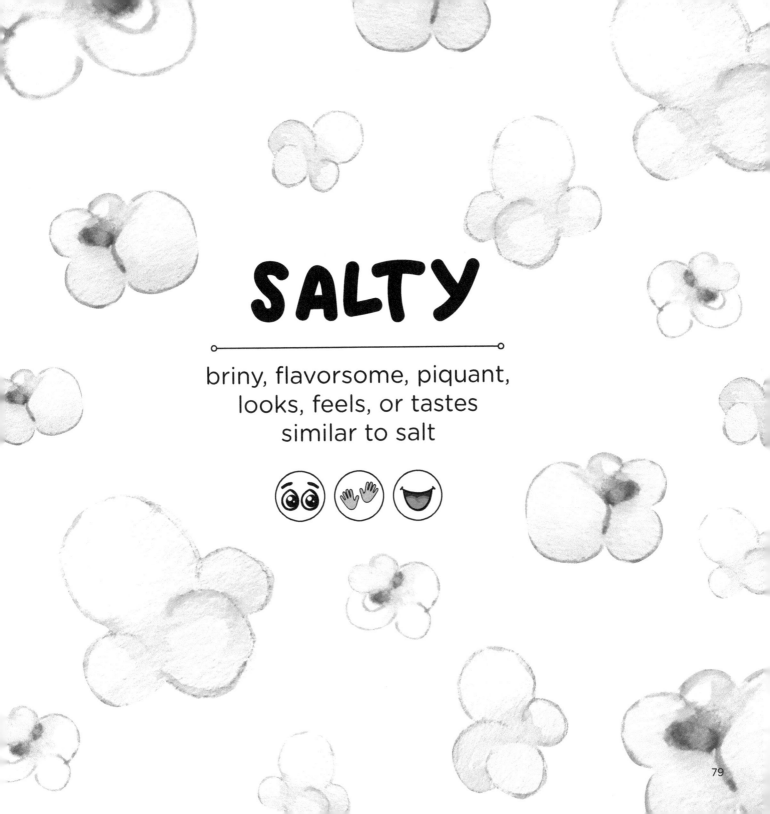

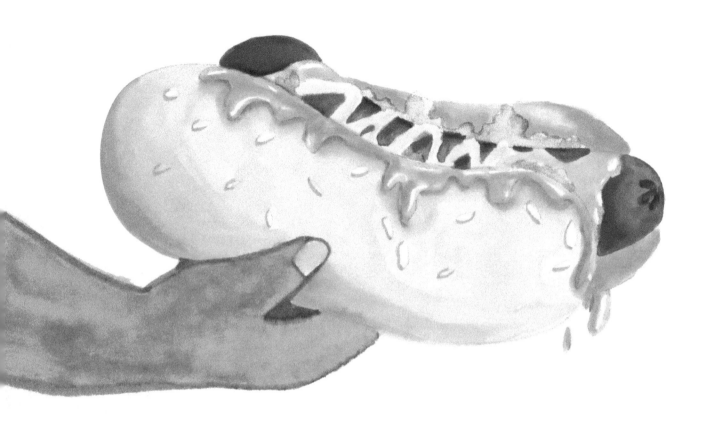

SAVORY

salty, spicy, well-seasoned,
free of sweetness

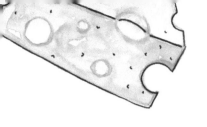
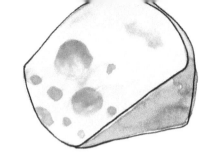
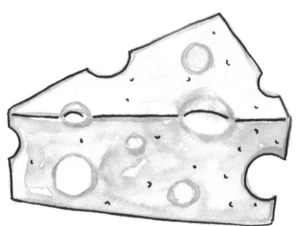
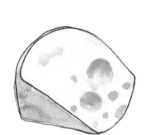
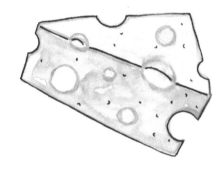

SHARP

bitter, pungent, tangy,
strong smell or taste

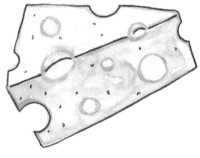
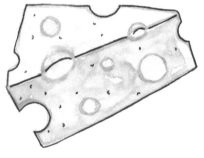
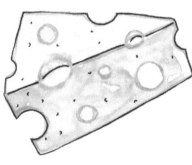
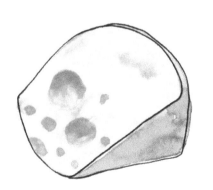
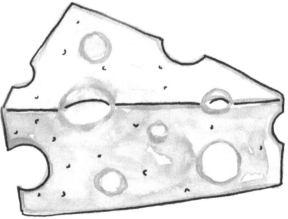
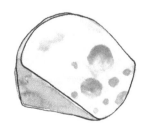
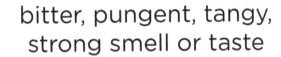
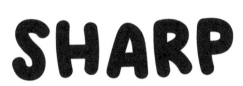

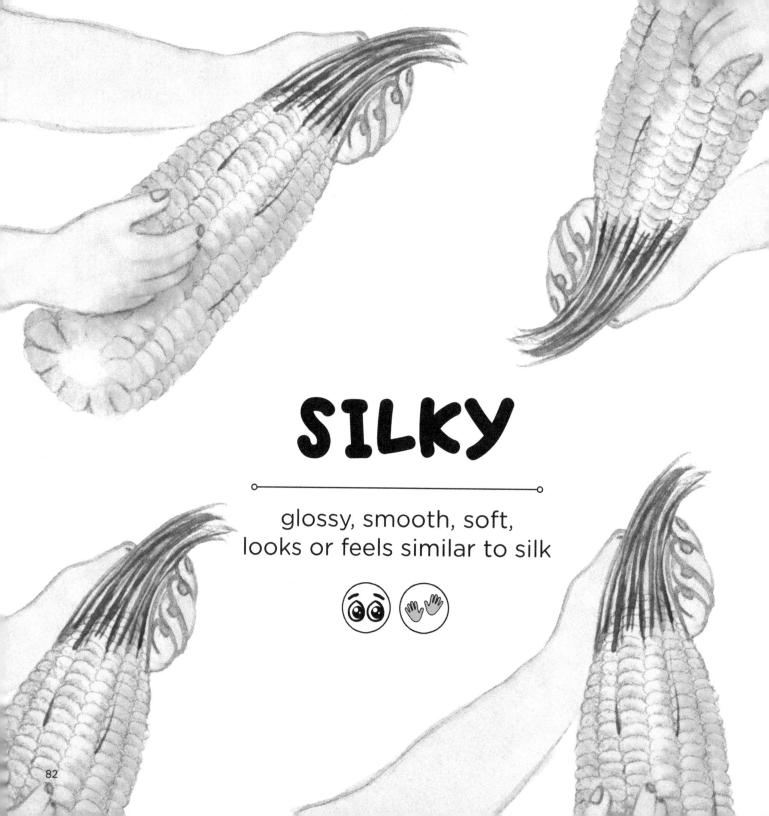

SILKY

glossy, smooth, soft,
looks or feels similar to silk

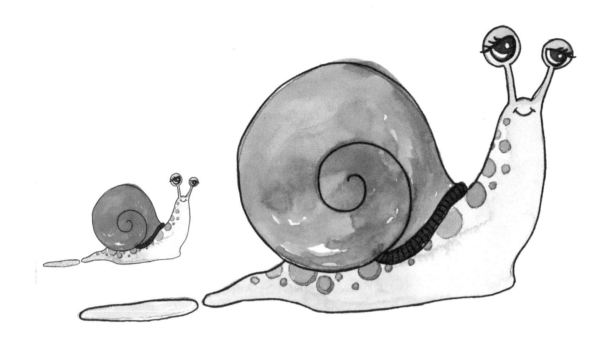

SLIMY

gooey, slippery, wet,
looks or feels similar to slime

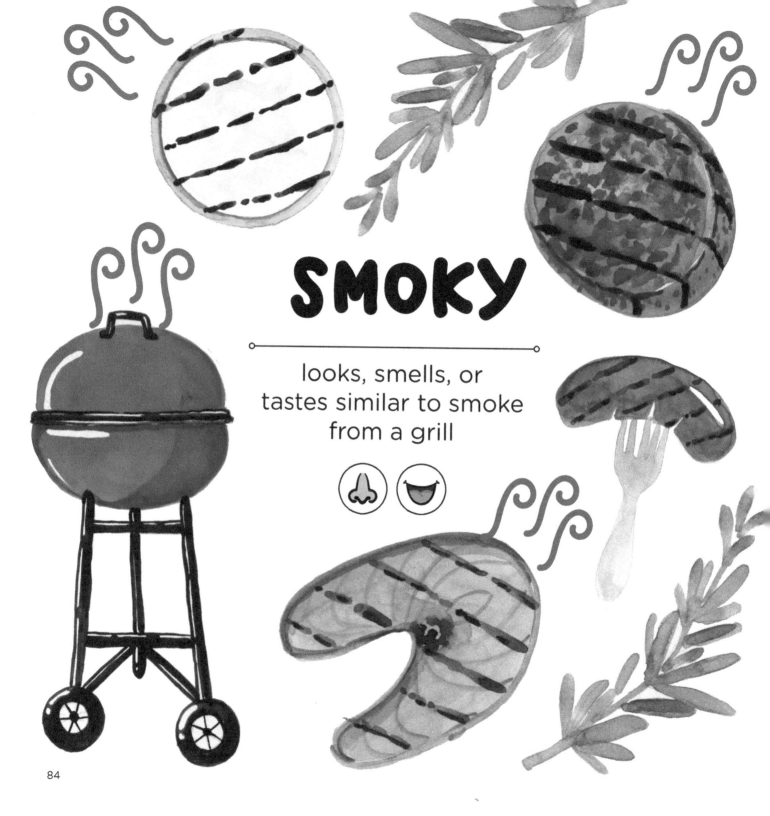

SMOKY

looks, smells, or
tastes similar to smoke
from a grill

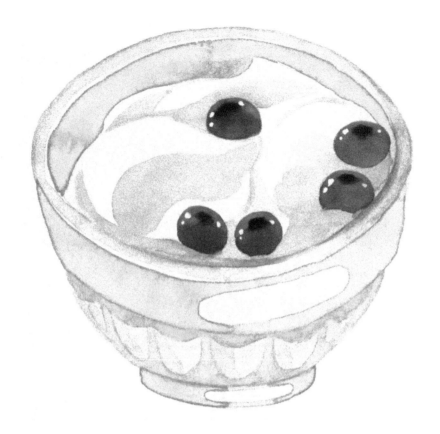

SMOOTH

○———————————○

even, flat, consistent texture

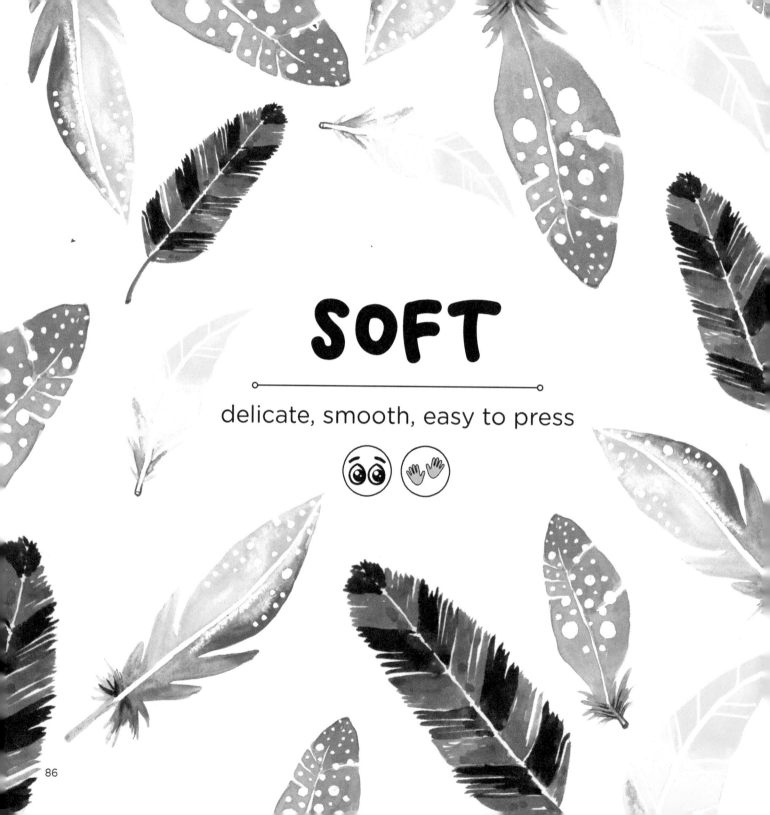

SOFT

delicate, smooth, easy to press

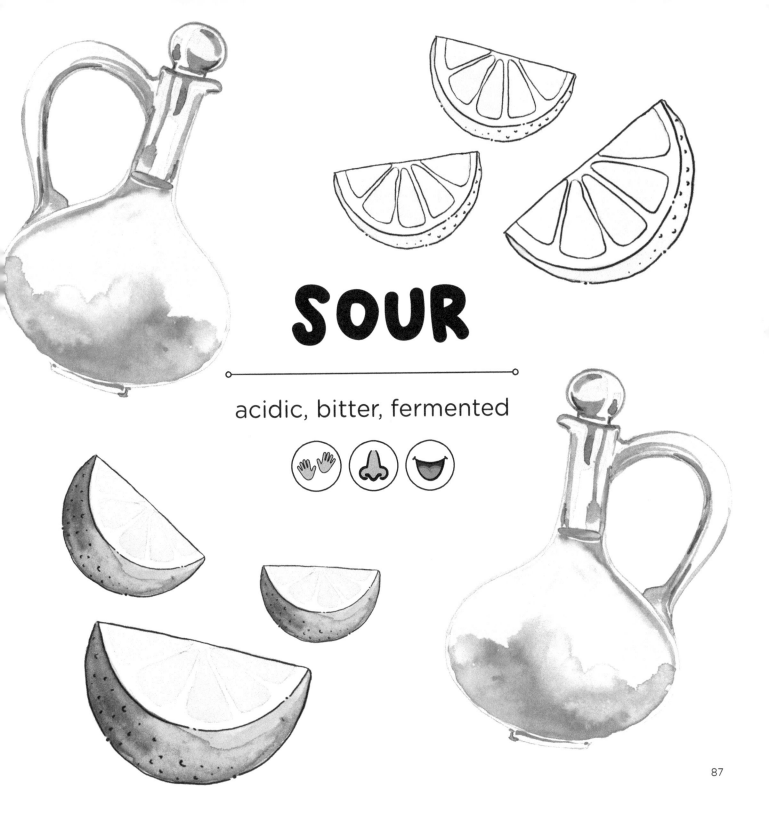

SOUR

acidic, bitter, fermented

SPICY

aromatic, hot,
strongly flavored

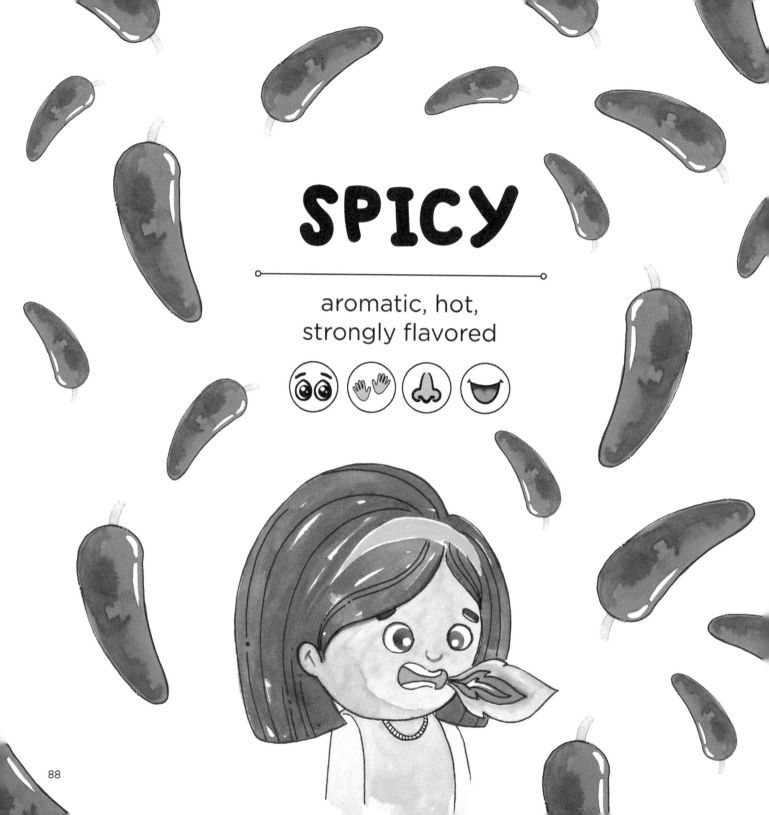

SPONGY

airy, light, soft,
looks or feels similar
to a sponge

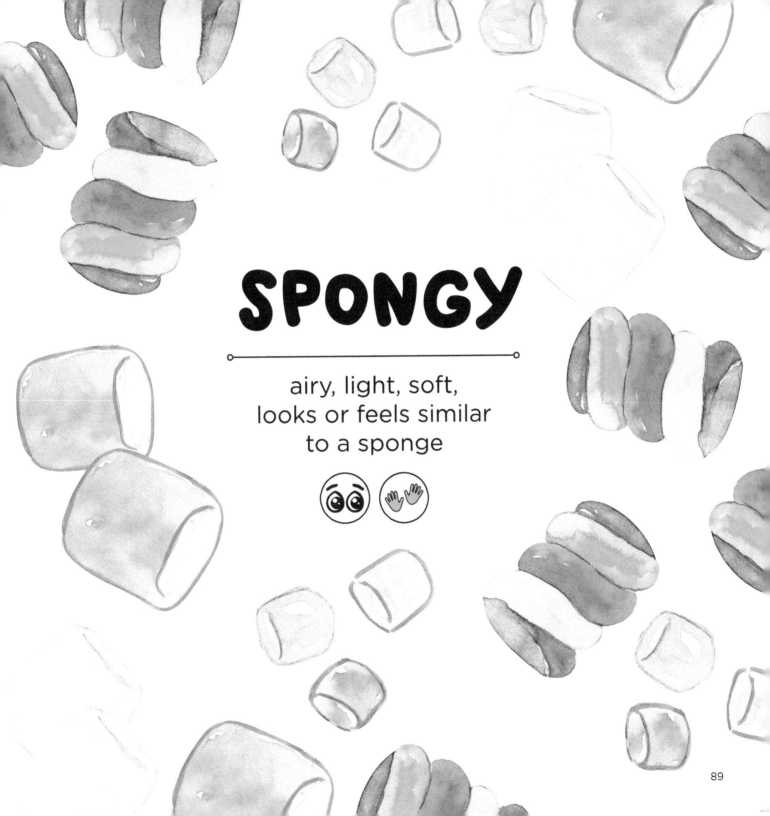

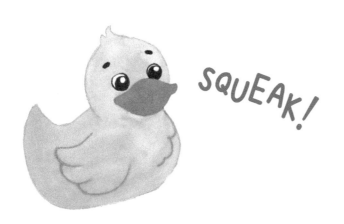

SQUEAK!

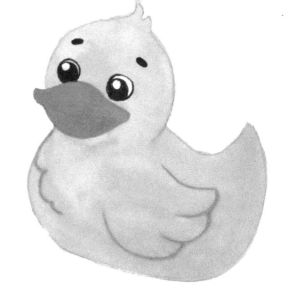

SQUEAK!

SQUEAKY

high-pitched, shrill, squeal

SQUEAK!

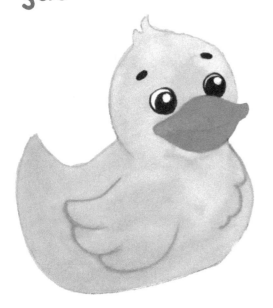

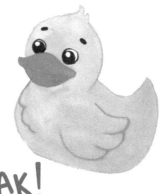

SQUEAK!

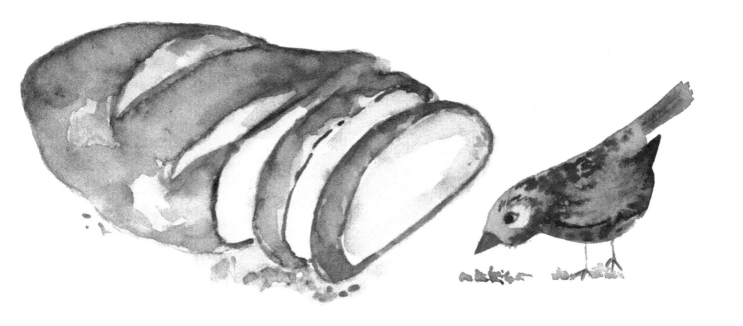

STALE

dry, old, musty, change
in appearance or texture

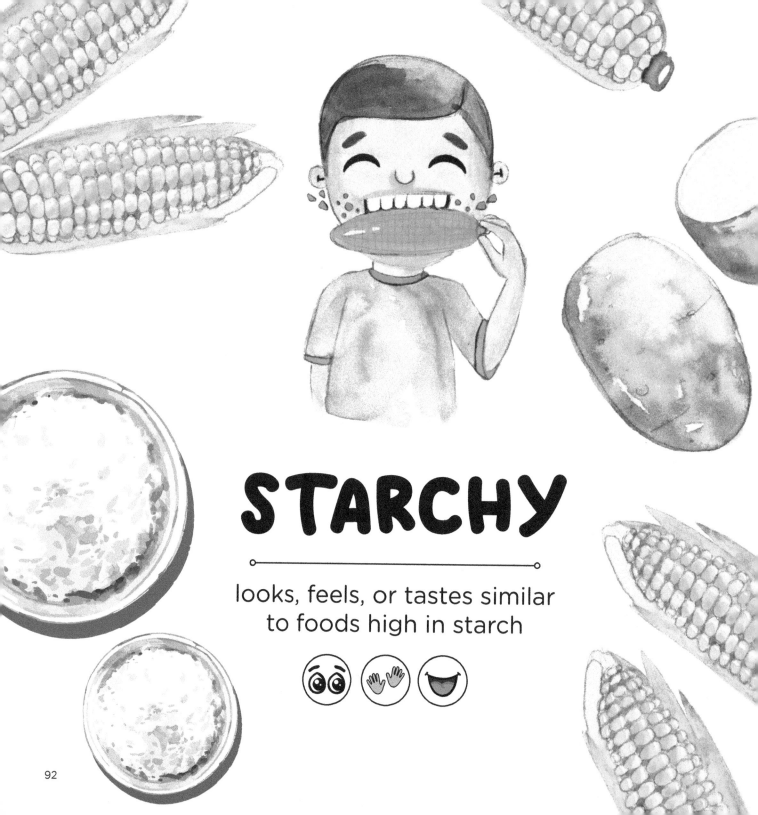

STARCHY

looks, feels, or tastes similar
to foods high in starch

92

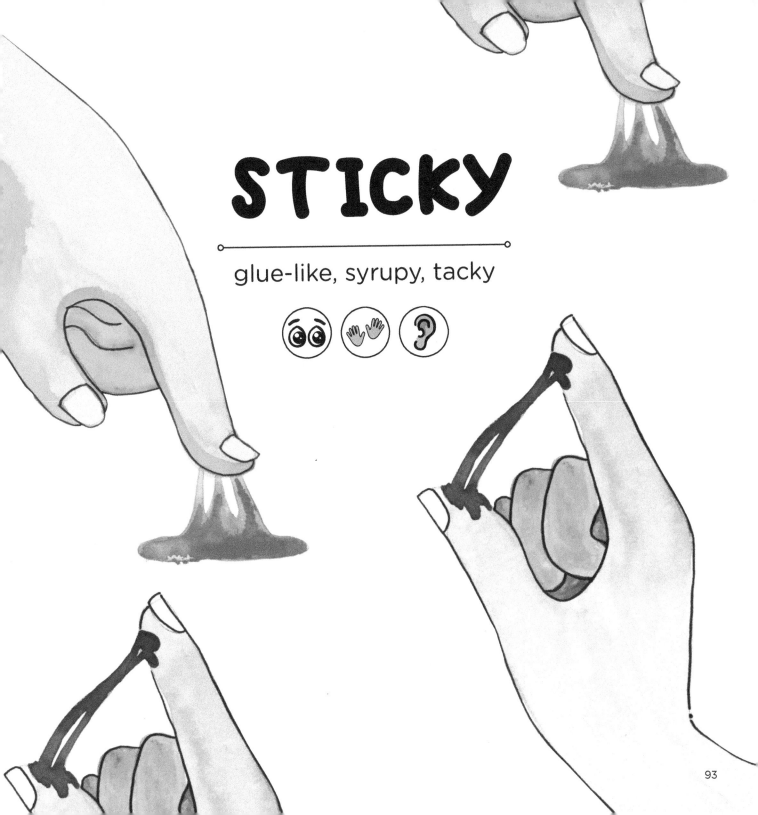

STICKY

glue-like, syrupy, tacky

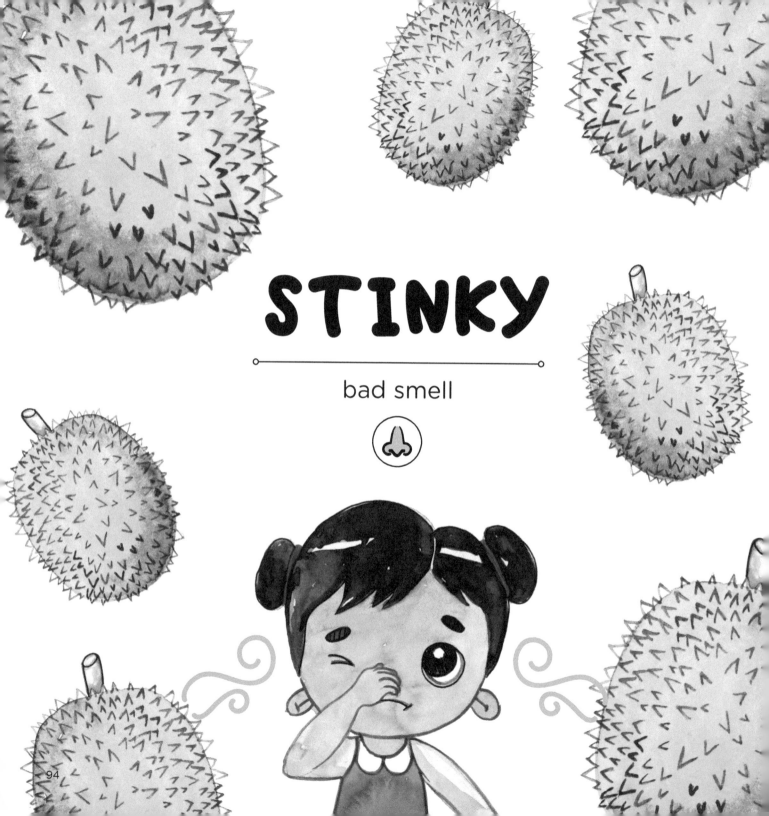

STINKY

bad smell

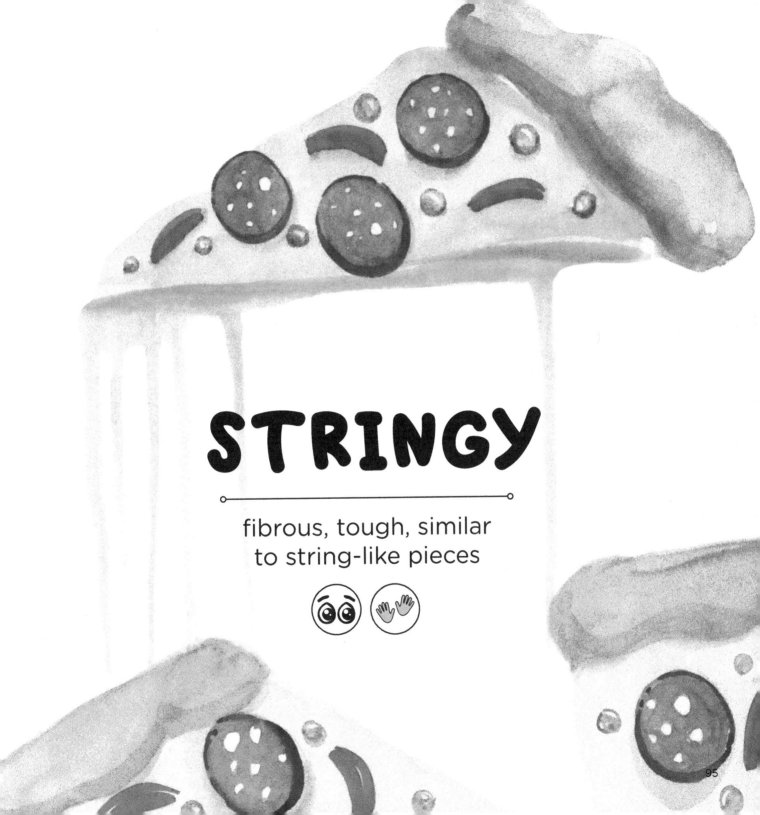

STRINGY

fibrous, tough, similar
to string-like pieces

SUBTLE

delicate, faint, light

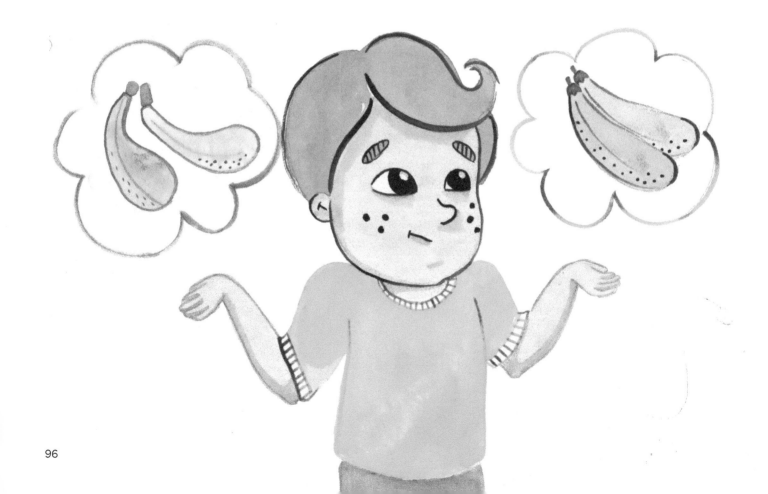

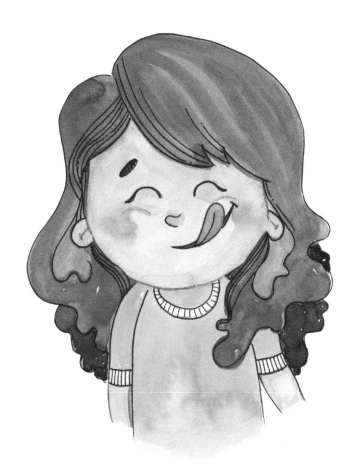

SUCCULENT

juicy, moist, yummy

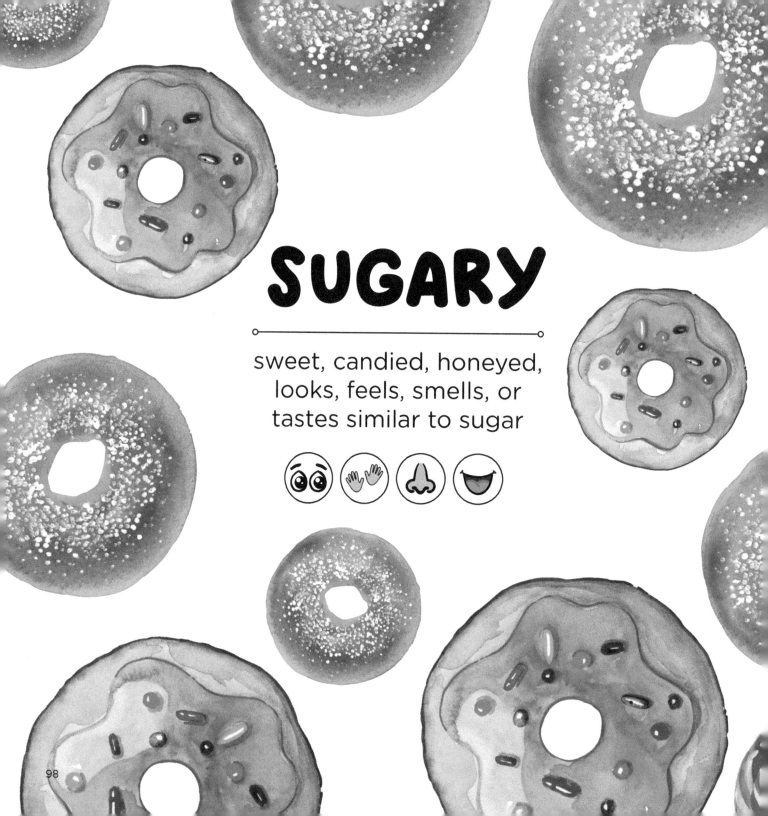

SUGARY

sweet, candied, honeyed, looks, feels, smells, or tastes similar to sugar

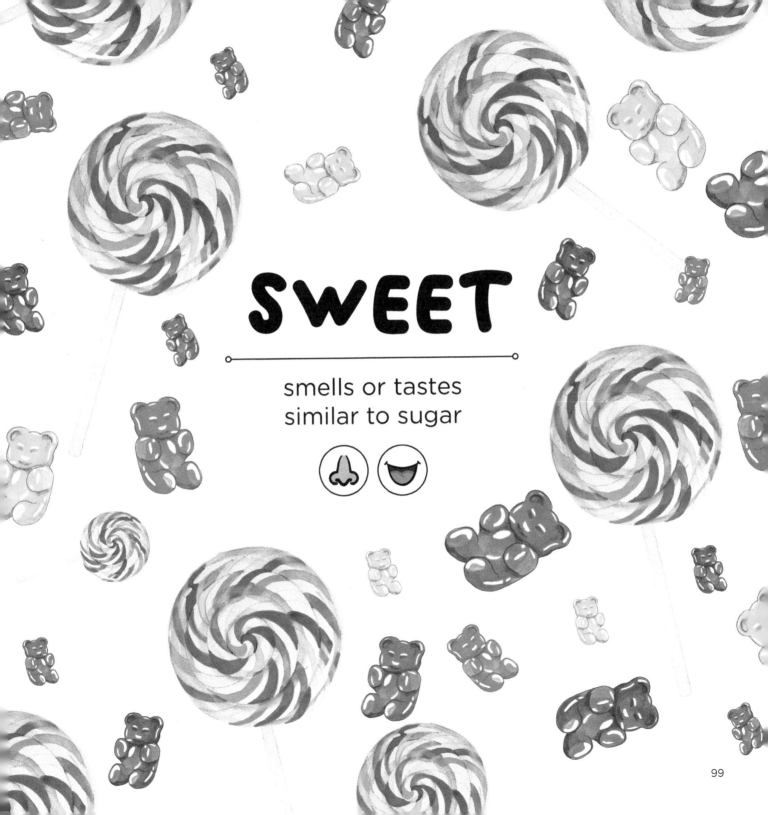

SWEET

smells or tastes
similar to sugar

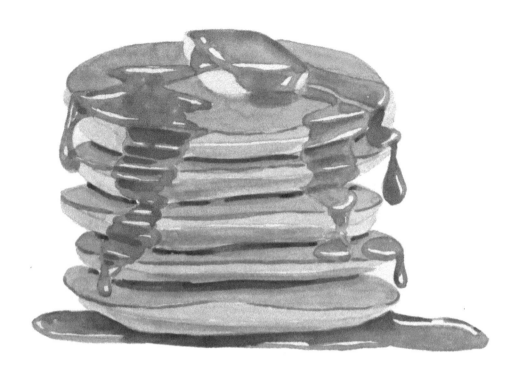

SYRUPY

sticky, sweet, thick,
looks, feels, smells, or tastes
similar to syrup

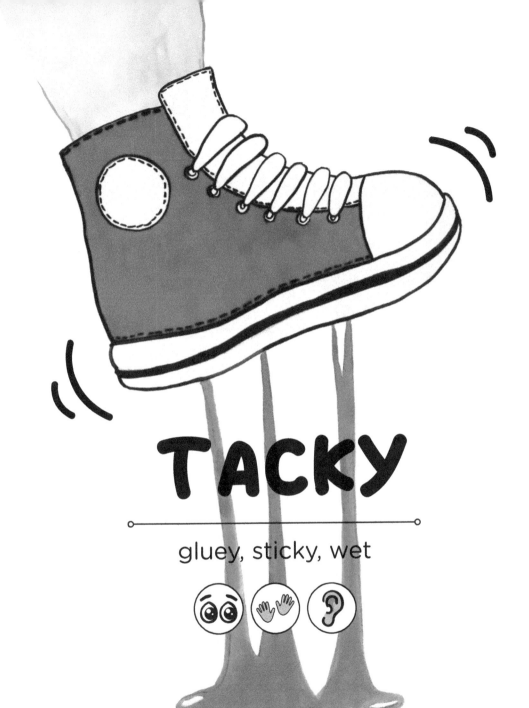

TACKY

gluey, sticky, wet

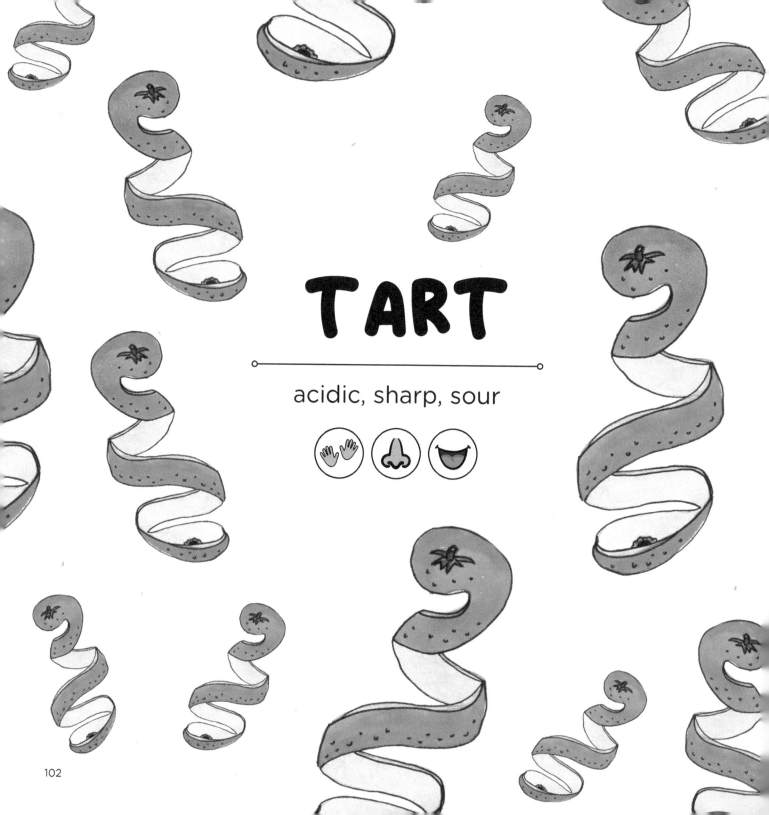

TART

acidic, sharp, sour

TASTELESS

bland, dull, flavorless

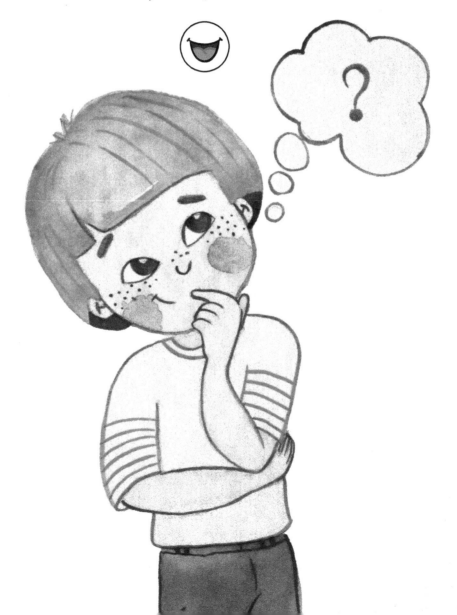

TENDER

delicate, soft,
easy to press

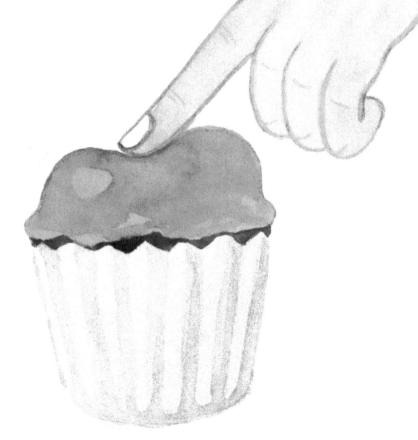

TEXTURED

bumpy, rough, uneven

TOUGH

dense, fibrous, hard

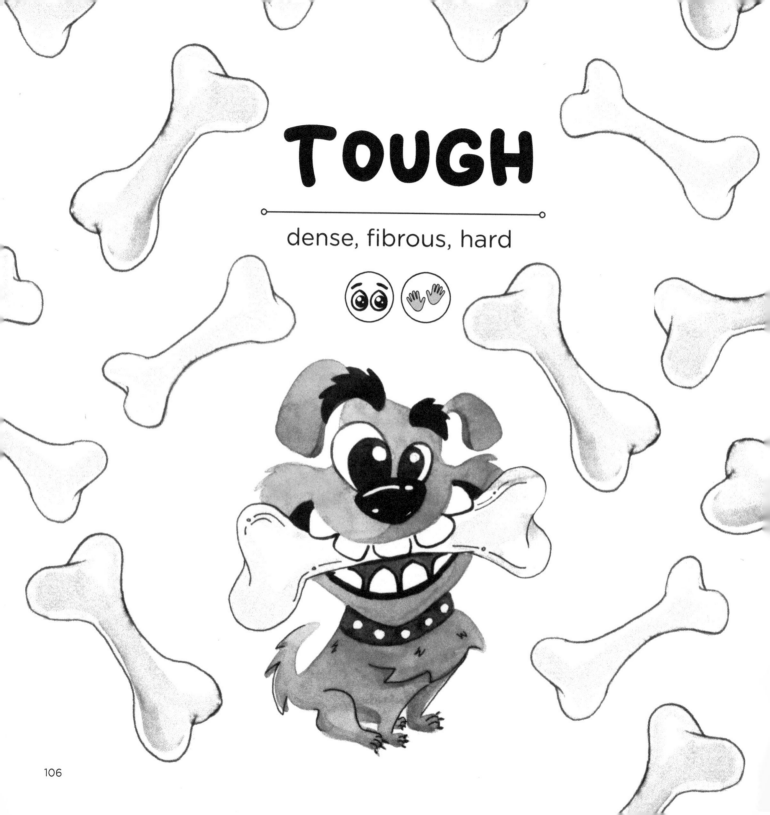

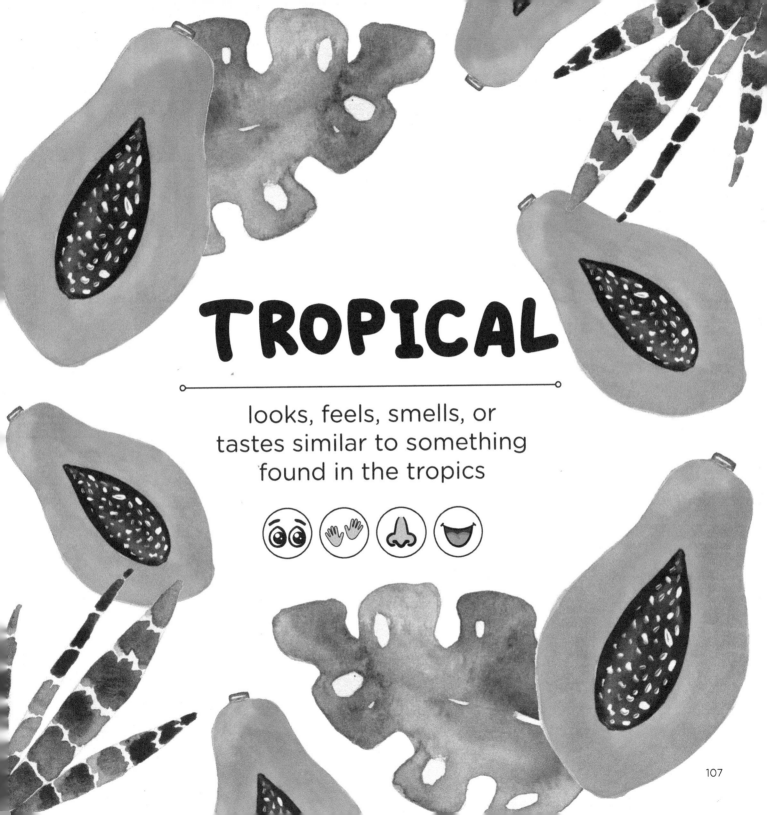

TROPICAL

looks, feels, smells, or
tastes similar to something
found in the tropics

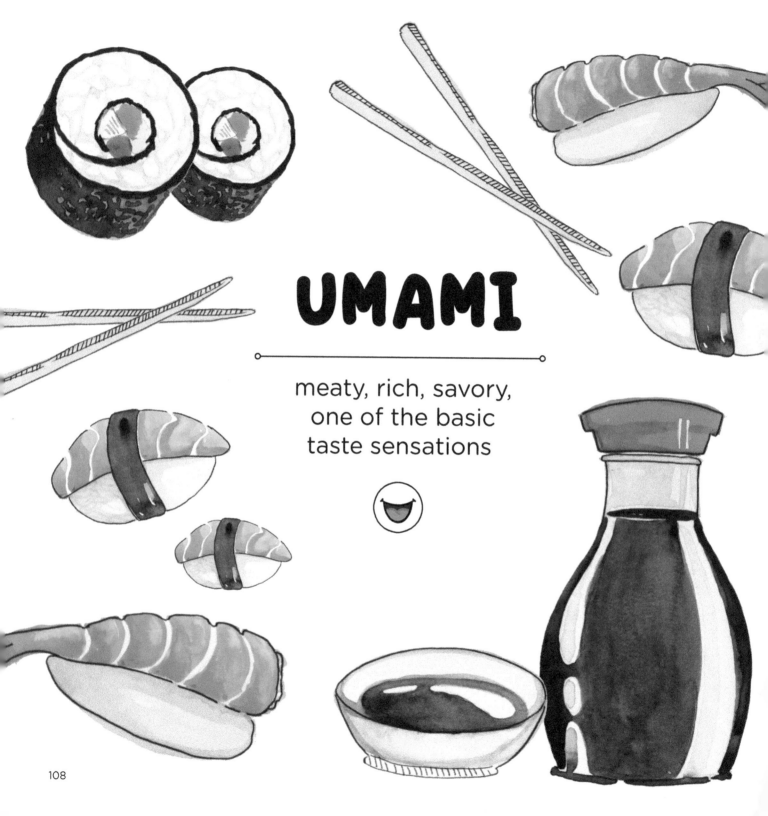

UMAMI

meaty, rich, savory,
one of the basic
taste sensations

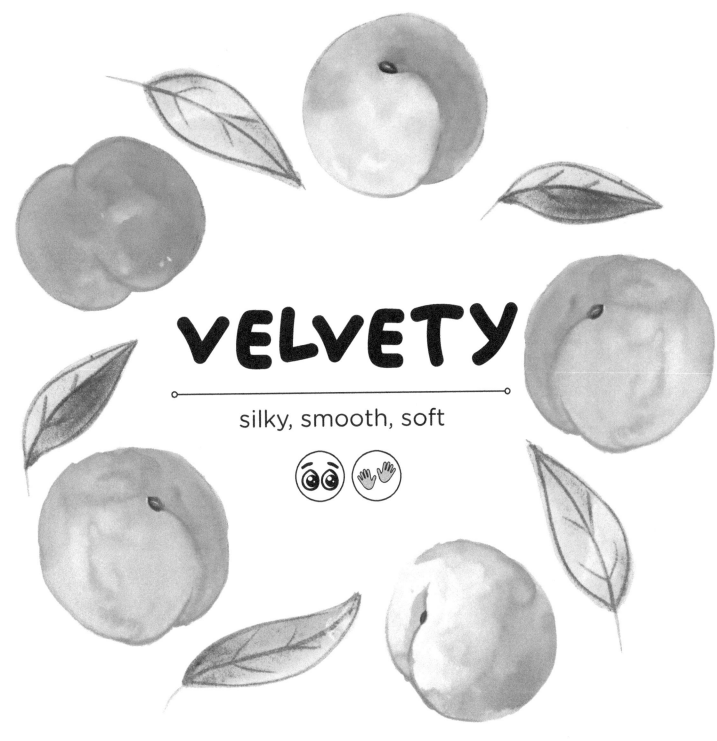

VELVETY

silky, smooth, soft

VIBRANT

bright, colorful, zippy

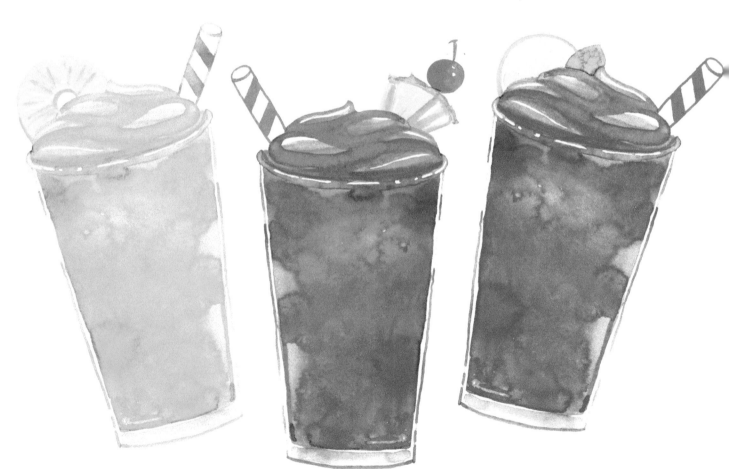

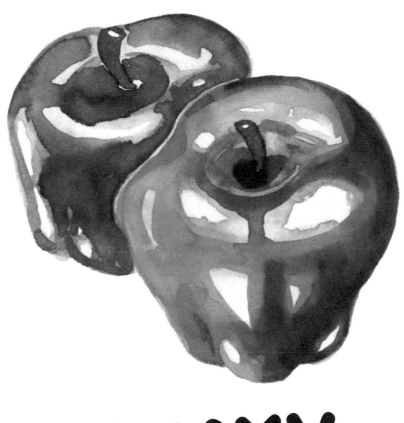

WAXY

---

shiny, smooth, sticky,
looks or feels similar to wax

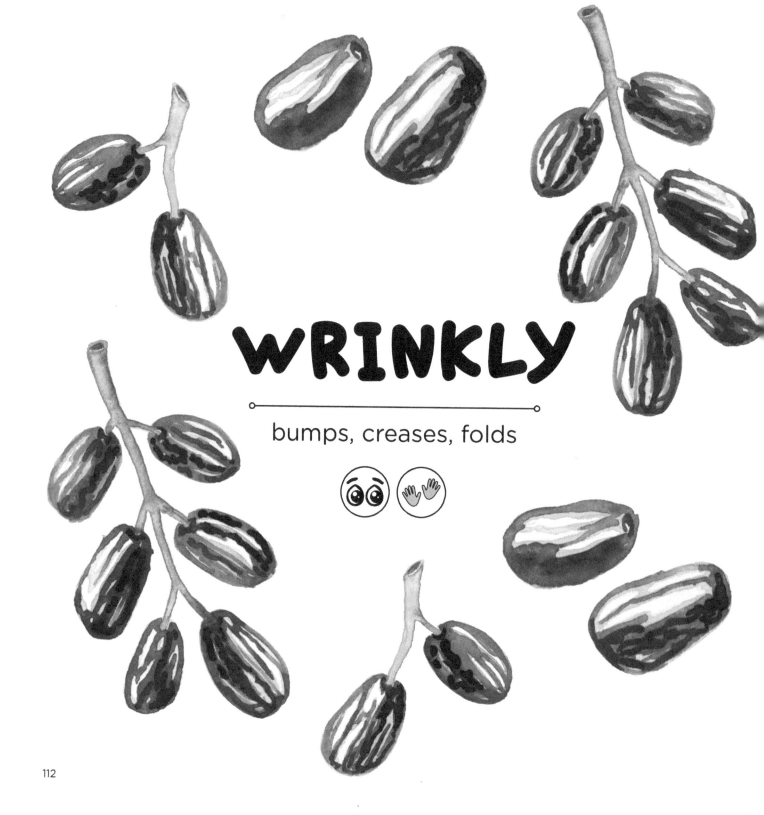

WRINKLY

bumps, creases, folds

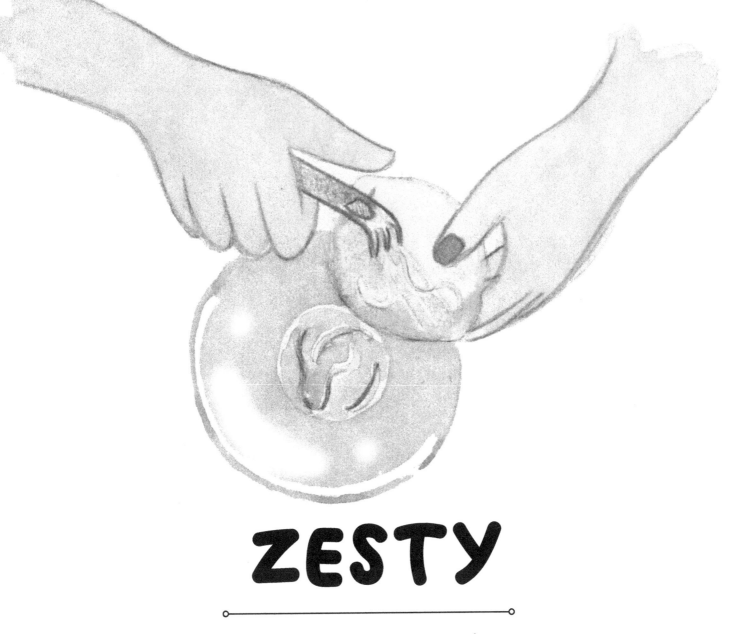

ZESTY

piquant, pungent, spicy

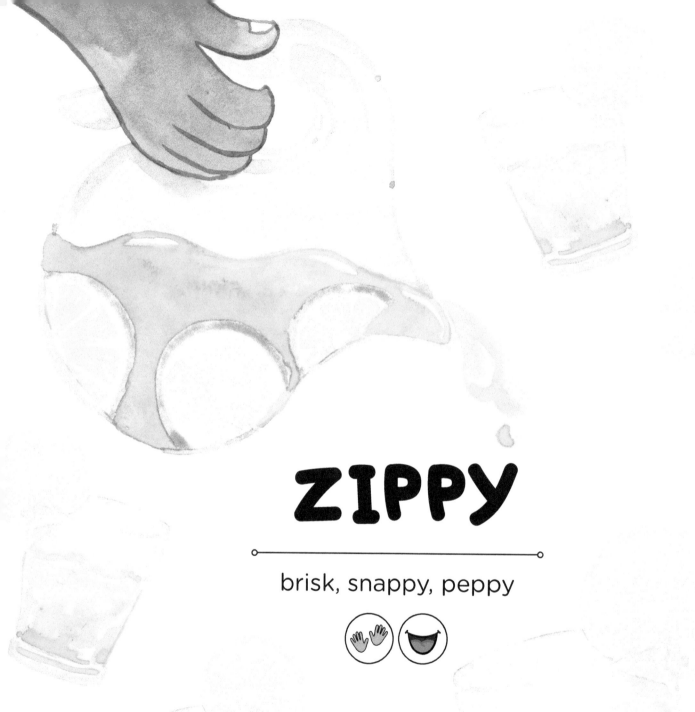

ZIPPY

brisk, snappy, peppy

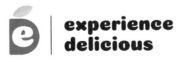

Lightning Source UK Ltd.
Milton Keynes UK
UKHW051023170720
366701UK00005B/135